EAT,
FAST,
SLIM

EAT, FAST, SLIM

The Life-Changing Fasting Diet
for Amazing Weight Loss and Optimum Health

AMANDA HAMILTON

DUNCAN BAIRD PUBLISHERS
LONDON

Eat, Fast, Slim
Amanda Hamilton

To my husband Crawfurd for holding the fort and holding my heart.

First published in the United Kingdom and Ireland in 2013 by
Duncan Baird Publishers,
an imprint of Watkins Publishing Limited
Sixth Floor, 75 Wells Street
London W1T 3QH

A member of Osprey Group

Managing Editor: Grace Cheetham
Editor: Jane McIntosh
Designer: Clare Thorpe
Production: Uzma Taj

A CIP record for this book is available from the British Library

ISBN: 978-1-84899-103-3

10 9 8 7 6 5 4 3 2 1

Typeset in Adobe Garamond Pro and
  Calluna Sans
Printed in the United Kingdom

Publisher's note: The information in this book is not intended as a substitute for professional medical advice and treatment. If you are pregnant or breastfeeding or have any special dietary requirements or medical conditions, it is recommended that you consult a medical professional before following any of the information or recipes contained in this book. Watkins Publishing Limited, or any other persons who have been involved in working on this publication, cannot accept responsibility for any errors or omissions, inadvertent or not, that may be found in the recipes or text, nor for any problems that may arise as a result of preparing one of these recipes or following the advice contained in this work.

Notes on the recipes
Unless otherwise stated
Use medium fruit and vegetables
Use fresh ingredients, including herbs
  and chillies
Do not mix metric and imperial
  measurements
1 tsp = 5ml 1 tbsp = 15ml 1 cup = 250ml

Glossary
Terms that appear in the Glossary appear in italics on first mention in the text.

CONTENTS

FOREWORD

We are all consuming more and doing less. The food we eat is higher in energy than ever, and we are eating more of it, more often. On average we are each taking in over 500 more calories a day than we did 30 years ago. Combine this with our increasingly sedentary lifestyles, and we have a recipe for weight gain and ill health.

In my practice I am already seeing the impact of this on my patients – and don't be lulled into thinking that this is just about the few unfortunate individuals at the extreme end of the scale who are the focus of various provocative TV documentaries on obesity. This is about the majority of the population. People with a normal body weight are now in the minority in the UK, with nearly two-thirds of us overweight or obese. And the implications for our health are enormous. Being overweight is not just about what dress size you take or being a bit "out of shape" – excess weight is a major risk factor for serious and even life-threatening conditions such as diabetes, heart disease and cancer.

But even these significant physical consequences underestimate the full impact that the rising tide of obesity is having. In my experience the damage done beneath the surface – shrinking self-esteem, ruined relationships and thwarted ambition – is equally destructive. The resulting mental health problems then perpetuate unhealthy habits in a vicious spiral that often feels impossible to break. The cost of obesity to the NHS is a staggering £5bn each year but the true financial impact of this epidemic in terms of the country's economic development is likely to be significantly higher. And, unlike most other outbreaks of disease, this tidal wave shows little sign of subsiding.

So, what is the solution? Well, contrary to popular belief the answer does not lie with the health service, government ministers or even the food industry – although of course they all play their part. It sits with each and every one of us. This is a collective problem with an individual solution. But where do we start? Almost every day we hear of some new diet plan or exercise regime – all making dramatic claims about how they will change our lives. Whilst each one may have some validity, the sheer volume of options feels bewildering, and with many of them giving conflicting advice who are we to believe? The resulting confusion fuels our apathy – we spend our time window shopping, absorbed in the theory of weight loss, perhaps trying a couple of dieting methods on for size and then, when nothing seems to happen immediately, we lose confidence in our own ability to change.

In *Eat, Fast, Slim* Amanda offers an antidote to our ambivalence. Through intermittent and juice fasting she has identified a method by which we can all reconnect with our bodies, moderate our food intake, increase our energy levels and become more active, healthy and happy as a result. By using this tried- and increasingly well-tested approach Amanda has seen significant changes in her own life and that of her clients. But, like all good scientists, Amanda also understands that her experience alone is not enough. Unlike so many other new health trends, Amanda makes no over-inflated claims regarding fasting, her approach is pragmatic and balanced – just like the diets she recommends. Throughout the book she draws upon the latest scientific evidence on fasting – giving her conclusions real credibility and allowing us all to be confident in the approach she recommends and the results it offers.

Amanda brings to the pages of this book an absolute wealth of knowledge and experience. She is not evangelical, there is no attempt to convince us or convert us – rather she is simply sharing with us what she has learned, empowering us with the information we need to make up our own minds, and offering us the tools we need to apply this approach to our lives should we wish to do so.

This book is an authentic account of many years of personal experience written by an inquisitive, rigorous healthcare practitioner with a clear understanding of the real world and the challenges we all face in our daily lives. It is incredibly timely, we all need to do something to rebalance the excesses of modern life and I, for one, am looking forward to giving it a go.

Dr Jonty Heaversedge
GP, author and broadcaster

LESS IS MORE

This is a book that I *had* to write. When I learned to fast, and how to harness the power of fasting, it challenged everything I'd ever read about how to eat, how to preserve health and how to stay in shape.

Fasting makes things really simple. It is scientifically proven to slow ageing and boost health and is something that every human being does instinctively, only most of us have forgotten how. Another "plus" is that fasting won't cost you anything – it's time rather than money that's needed. The techniques that inspired modern day fasting might well date back millennia but fasting has never been more needed than right here, right now.

In this book I will be providing persuasive arguments in favour of fasting, backed up by scientific research, and plenty of practical advice. Don't worry, though – I'm not a finger-wagging, matron type. I know that healthy habits must be fun in order to be achievable in the long term so all the science is presented alongside a hefty dose of real life.

When you first get into fasting, it can be hard to figure out which technique will suit you best so I'll help you to navigate your way through the fasting world. **Broadly speaking, there are the intermittent fasts (what I call *lifestyle* fasts) and juice fasts although, increasingly, fasts are becoming known according to their duration in hours or days – 16/8, 5/2, alternate day and so on.** Most are do-able even for someone with only a faint whiff of interest in healthy living, but some require caution. In this book I only feature the techniques that make the grade in terms of scientifically referenced benefits and practical application.

I will also explain why men and women should approach fasting differently, and how best to use fasting for fat loss. I'll tell you how to use fasting to enhance mental and physical performance, and explain how even subtle changes in eating habits can prolong your life.

But before we begin, let me share a little story with you – after all, the idea of learning not to eat, rather than advice on *what* to eat, might sound a bit ridiculous coming from someone who has made a career as a nutritionist!

When I first started working with fasting after learning the technique during a trip to India (more about that later), I couldn't explain the dramatic results I was experiencing – it all seemed like a happy accident. News of my success with fasting spread by word of mouth and soon there was a steady stream of customers in my nutrition clinic. I knew I was onto something really special and that when I'd acted on "gut" feelings in the past, things had turned out well... and so I ended up following my dream by moving to Spain to set up a juice detox retreat based on fasting. I quite literally moved my entire life and worldly belongings to a one-donkey town in the mountains of Andalusia.

Indeed, most of my friends thought it was either an early mid-life crisis (I was only 27 years old) or there was a man involved. Neither was true. I simply believe that fortune favours the brave and I felt utterly compelled to follow the idea through to fruition. One year later, my fasting retreat became the subject of a reality television show that documented the incredible results. It ended up being shown in 22 countries around the world – and the rest, as they say, is history. If that isn't incredible enough, listen to what happened next...

A decade on from this venture into the unknown (having become a wife and mother to a blended family of four children in the meantime), I decided to write a book to explain why fasting works so well. I took the opportunity of starting my formal research during some time-out at one of the spas where I run my retreats.

I curled up in my chair to read about the history of fasting, and as I worked through the first chapter I realized I was in the spa founded by the medical expert, Stanley Leif, who first introduced fasting programmes to Britain between the First and Second World Wars. Not only that, I was sitting in the only room in the 80-bedroom spa that had his name on the door. Stanley Leif died in 1972 and, yes, it felt like he was there in the room.

In a nutshell, here is why learning to fast was life-changing for me and why I think you should give it a go:

- Fasting shifted my last annoying 4.5kg (10lb) in weight, without me having to obsess about counting calories or following ridiculous "fad diets".

- Fasting is good for me on the inside and makes me look better on the outside. When something makes you feel this good, it is easy to stick with it.

- Fasting makes me feel emotionally in control (and a little virtuous).

- Fasting gets my hunger under control.

- Ever since I discovered fasting, according to the most accurate test available my biological age has remained a full decade younger than what it says on my passport, and this is in spite of having given birth to two children. I'm not showing off – it just works!

Amanda

INTRODUCTION

THE BENEFITS OF FASTING

Fasting is not something that most of us ever think about – food is everywhere and in all likelihood right now you're within striking distance of an emergency skinny latte and a muffin. Now I love food as much as the next person, so **what I find great about fasting is that it's as much about eating delicious things as it is about abstaining**. And there are none of the harmful effects you get from following crazy diets or popping pills, because **fasting provides a natural high, an inner boost that works with your body, not against it**.

When I first learned about fasting, it was in the context of an invitation to join an intensive meditation retreat in the Himalayas. In fact, I only stumbled across meditation in a foggy, end-of-yoga-class kind of way (and usually ended up snoring!). By contrast, I'd always been fascinated by the inner poise of people who did yoga. I didn't just envy their lithe bodies – I wanted their unshakable contentment and smiling eyes. How did they manage to waft around so effortlessly and have boundless energy for eye-watering yoga moves? And they all seemed to look incredibly youthful and naturally glowing. What was their secret? Whatever it was, I had to have it. So, as you do when you are childless and too young to care about a job and responsibilities, I gave up a regular salary and sold my worldly possessions to enjoy an alternative (and rather late) gap year in an Indian ashram where I planned to study yoga and meditation. Admittedly, it was the thought of becoming supple and slender rather than discovering nirvana that sweetened the deal for me. As it happened, one of the simplest techniques I learned over those intensive months has become one of my most important life lessons for mind and body – how to fast.

Like a lot of things that are amazingly good for you, such as yoga, fasting has been around for donkey's years. Most of the major faiths around the world incorporate some form of fasting within their religious practice. So whilst fasting might sound shocking to those indoctrinated by the mantra of breakfast, lunch and dinner, it was a way of life for our Palaeolithic ancestors, and even now it's something that yogis and millions of people of the Muslim, Mormon and Jewish faiths do regularly. **My version of fasting, however, has got nothing to do with religion. It's true that fasting often brings clarity of mind but, as I hope you'll discover for yourself, it's what it does to the body that's truly extraordinary.**

Fasting adds years to your life and life to your years. It's undoubtedly an excellent way of shifting the pounds and can help to change your shape. But, as you'll discover, it helps your body work better on the inside, too. One of the amazing *proven* side-effects of fasting is that it's anti-ageing at a cellular level, which is the only place that really counts. This inside-out approach really can help to create a glowing beauty from within. This is because fasting gives your body a break and a chance to catch up on its inner "to-do list". By allowing your body to have more of what it needs and less of what it doesn't, you put less strain on your body's resources and have more time to do the maintenance.

Fasting is so easy, you really can't fail. In fact, it's something we all do already – *breakfast*, quite literally, is breaking a fast of around 12 hours. And let's not forget one of the best things of all – if you "do" fasting properly (there are several techniques to choose from and by the end of the book you will discover which one suits you), **you can finally give up on the endless hamster wheel of weight loss**

and gain that sees otherwise sane and successful people becoming slaves to whatever dieting fad happens to be the flavour of the month. I know the pain of that world because I existed in it for so long. I also know how good it feels to be free of it.

FASTING VERSUS OTHER WEIGHT-LOSS APPROACHES

It's time to stick my neck out. I'd go as far to say that **I see fasting as the future of weight loss**. The diet industry is just that – an industry – and a great many consumers have woken up to the fact that they have been sold a dummy. As any seasoned dieter knows, behind the hype and celebrity following, many trendy diet plans are just plain silly and impractical.

Long-term calorie restriction, the backbone of traditional weight loss, can make you prone to weight gain. Not only that, the nutritional aspects of many commercially savvy weight-loss plans are at best borderline, and at worst downright dangerous. The fact that one of the largest dieting companies in the world is owned by a confectionery company illustrates (to me at least) that the industry behind dieting and the promise of weight loss may need a bit of a shake-up.

Fundamentally, fasting for weight loss is all about nutrition. When you *do* eat, you must eat well. When you're fasting, there's no cutting out of major food groups such as carbohydrates or essential fats. In this book you'll find lots of information about what to eat when you adopt a fasting regime, rather than simply calculating when you don't eat. In fact, nutrition is even more important when you're fasting since you're eating less overall.

If I'm right and fasting becomes the next big thing in dieting, what will happen? Well, fasting is already rapidly gaining in popularity and when a trend begins – particularly a global trend

– newspaper headlines don't necessarily get all the facts right. And when a trend imbibes the collective consciousness, particularly in weight loss, you can guarantee that money-wasting gimmicks will follow. Therefore, as part of your induction into the world of fasting, I'll be giving you a gimmick-free tour of the scientifically backed benefits of fasting for weight loss, longevity and performance.

Every piece of advice in this book is sound and practical. In my research I've discovered that in order to achieve the best results, **fasting techniques should be subtly different for women and men, and different again if you're using fasting to enhance performance.** Whilst science acts as the perfect signpost, we're all unique – biologically, physically and emotionally, and ultimately it remains your job and your job alone to turn evidence into action.

Even with the greatest advances, there are certain things that science, or nutrition for that matter, can't explain fully but I will nevertheless attempt to describe how **fasting may make you feel more connected and happier in yourself.** Fasting, more than any other nutrition or diet approach, can help you to reset your attitude and recognize the difference between physical hunger and appetite. Slowing down your eating can make the experience as much a "mental break" as a physical boost. Indeed, fasting has been used for centuries as a method of mental and spiritual purification. It's like setting a part of you free again.

THE SCIENCE ON FASTING

The scientific studies on fasting focus largely on alternate-day fasting and on prolonged periods of fasting. Much of the scientific research is done on animals rather than on humans – mainly because it's considered unethical to starve people for no reason! However, the evidence that is out there about the benefits of fasting is just so compelling and exciting that it's worthy of a few minutes of your attention (and I'll be busting several dieting myths along the way).

The following are a few highlights from the science of fasting that we'll explore in the forthcoming chapters:

FASTING FOR WEIGHT LOSS

- It might seem counter-intuitive, but intermittent fasting could help you get your hunger under control. This is partly because of its effects on your hunger hormones, and partly because it helps you to learn the difference between physical and emotional hunger.

- Forget what you've been told about regular meals boosting metabolism – studies show that people who are overweight tend to snack *more* often.

- Fasting is just as effective as traditional diets for losing weight, but might be easier to stick to and less likely to slow your metabolism – perfect if you want to lose that last bit of stubborn flesh.

- If you're stressed, and troubled by weight around your middle, shorter fasts may be better at tackling belly fat than longer ones.

FASTING FOR HEALTH

- Fasting – especially in combination with eating less protein – acts like a "spring clean" for the body by switching on a cellular mechanism called *autophagy* and by reducing the levels of a hormone called *insulin-like growth factor (IGF-1)* that can send cell growth out of control.

- Regular juice fasts may deliver potent anti-ageing benefits without you having to cut out food completely.

- Whichever fasting format you choose, it's likely to reduce inflammation – good news for conditions such as eczema, asthma and arthritis.

- Contrary to the popular belief that sugary snacks are "brain food", fasting may help adults to concentrate better. It could even help to build new brain cells.

FASTING FOR WOMEN AND FOR MEN
- The effects on blood sugar control seem to be different in women and men. Studies suggest that fasting improves men's blood sugar control, but may not have a beneficial effect on women's.

- Most women know that adopting any new healthy habit is generally more challenging the week before their period starts. So my advice is to go easy that week. Your nearest and dearest will be thankful too.

- For a woman, the best time to try fasting is a few days after the start of a period. Once you're used to it, fasting could help to quash PMS cravings.

- When it comes to the overall impact of fasting on menstrual cycles, we only have animal studies to go on, and the effects aren't clear. However, any improvements in overall diet usually go some way to helping with any menstrual problems – so make sure you pay as much attention to what you do eat as you do to what you don't eat. If you notice any negative changes, or have lost weight to the point where your periods become disrupted, stop fasting.

FASTING FOR GYM BUNNIES

- Doing weight training while fasting can help your body build more muscle.

- If you favour cardio workouts, training while fasting can help your body learn to tap into its fat stores more intensively – but it's not such a good idea to run a race without eating beforehand.

- Again, there are gender differences – men tend to build muscle so long as they work out before their main meal, whereas women seem to respond better to training after a meal.

HOW TO USE THIS BOOK

The book is split into four parts. It's designed to give you an overview of the history and science of fasting, but more importantly there's lots of practical information to help you make fasting work for you. Whether you're simply interested in finding out a bit more about fasting, are contemplating giving it a try, or are already a regular faster looking for meal ideas and support, there's something here for you.

THE SECRETS, SCIENCE AND INCREDIBLE BENEFITS OF FASTING

Here's where we get into the science and benefits of fasting. You'll learn about my own experiences with fasting, and read the stories of people who have successfully used fasting to improve health conditions, lose weight, and get fitter. You can read it all in one go, or dip into the topics that interest you most.

MAKING FASTING WORK FOR YOU

In this section, you'll learn how to make fasting work for you and your lifestyle and discover the things you should think through before getting started. I'll help you decide which method will suit you best, from a short-term juice fast to a twice-weekly low-calorie day, to skipping one meal a day. You'll also learn how to get into the right state of mind to begin your first fast.

PUTTING FASTING INTO PRACTICE

This is where we get really practical. I'll provide you with lots of useful information on exercise and nutrition. After all, one of the most important messages you'll hear throughout the book is that when you *do* eat, you must eat well. Here, I also detail what to expect on your first fast and when fasting simply isn't a good idea.

FASTING PLANS AND RECIPES

And finally, here you will find day-by-day plans and delicious, nutritious recipes that make fasting as easy as possible!

PART 1

THE SECRETS, SCIENCE AND INCREDIBLE BENEFITS OF FASTING

- FOLLOWERS OF FASTING
- EAT, FAST AND LOSE WEIGHT
- EAT, FAST AND LIVE LONGER
- EAT, FAST AND PERFORM BETTER

CHAPTER 1

FOLLOWERS OF FASTING

FASTING THROUGH HISTORY

Fasting simply means extending the time between meals when we don't eat, and is something that humans have practised since they first walked the planet. It's only in recent times that we've had access to food 24 hours a day. Before then, we typically went for extended periods without eating. **Fasting's no passing "fad" – unlike the modern trend of "grazing", the notion that we should constantly be ingesting small amounts.** Interest in when and what we eat and drink has been increasing steadily and is set to continue. Nutritional knowledge helps us understand how our bodies and minds work, and nutritional intervention has a major role to play in the lives of everyone, from Olympic athletes to busy mums and people with medical conditions. No longer seen as something "alternative", nutritional therapy has now gone mainstream.

THE ANCIENT GREEKS
The Ancient Greeks were great believers in fasting. Spiritual masters such as **Pythagoras** (c.575–c.495BCE) are known not to have admitted any students to the higher levels of their teaching unless they had first "purified" themselves through fasting. The philosopher **Plato** (c.429–c.347BCE) said that he fasted for greater mental and physical efficiency, as did his pupil **Aristotle** (c.384–c.322BCE).

Hippocrates (c.460–c.377BCE), effectively one of the founders of modern medicine, realized the role of fasting in weight loss:

"...those desiring to lose weight should perform hard work before food. Meals should be taken after exertion and while still panting from fatigue. They should, moreover, only eat once per day."

He also made the observation:

"Everyone has a physician inside him or her; we just have to help it in its work. The natural healing force within each one of us is the greatest force in getting well. Our food should be our medicine. But to eat when you are sick is to feed your sickness."

Hippocrates believed that the bulk of diseases are caused by "autointoxication" and that fasting gives the body the chance to "repose" and auto-generate – in other words, to get a much-needed rest for the digestive organs to recover. For illnesses and fevers in the "acute crisis stage", he prescribed a strict fast with nothing but supportive water or medicinal teas, or a very light juice cleanse. The physician **Galen** (c.130–c.210CE) also advocated fasting for his patients, and the philosopher **Plutarch** (c.46–c.120CE) took a similar view:

"Instead of using medicine, rather, fast a day."

AYURVEDA

The Hindu system of traditional medicine, Ayurveda, has been popular in India for 2,500 years. Ayurveda teaches that light fasting stimulates the digestive fire (*agni* in Sanskrit), which in turn burns your body's fuel more efficiently, producing less toxic waste (*ama*).

In Ayurvedic medicine, a fast is considered an effective way to cleanse accumulated toxins from the body and mind, improve clarity and increase energy. If you were to try an Ayurvedic-style fast, you would fast once a week using salt-free liquids, such as fresh vegetable juice, water, yogurt mixed with water and cumin powder, or milk boiled with spices such as ginger.

Similar to the practice in juice-fasting retreats in spas all over Europe and the USA, Ayurvedic fasting is often combined with a detoxification programme (*panchakarma*) where supportive therapies are customized for an individual's constitution, age, physical health, immune status and a host of other factors. Even though juice fasting retreats and body builders may claim the science of fasting as their own, they owe much to Ayurveda and, more recently, the fields of natural hygiene, nature cure and naturopathy, all of which use fasting as a core treatment in healing.

These healing traditions, ancient and modern, have one thing in common – they support the body to heal itself, rather than turning to medicines or to invasive treatment to treat illness or create positive change. In Germany, fasting is even referred to as "awakening the physician within". Indeed, there's a wealth of historic and emerging research that we'll draw on in this book to illustrate the value and efficacy of fasting as a therapeutic and valuable medical intervention.

Learning to work with this natural approach can take just as long as learning a conventional medical approach. For example, in India, training to become an Ayurvedic doctor takes five years of study – as long as it takes to become a medical doctor in the UK – and, in the USA, naturopaths are now able to qualify to doctorate level.

POETRY AND PROSE

There are a mind-boggling number of faiths and religions that have a version of fasting within their sacred texts. These include but are not limited to Sikhism, Baha'i, Judaism, Jainism, Hinduism, Mormonism, Christianity, Greek Orthodox, Catholicism, Taoism, Buddhism and Islam. Unsurprisingly, given this historic role of fasting in many faiths and civilizations as a means of achieving spiritual awakening, fasting has inspired a number of works of poetry and prose, the best known of which is from the 13th-century Persian Muslim poet and Sufi mystic Mawlana Jalaluddin Rumi (1207–1273), better known simply as Rumi. His poems have been widely translated throughout the world and in 2007 he was voted the most popular poet in America. Here's one of his poems:

"There's hidden sweetness in the stomach's emptiness.
We are lutes, no more, no less. If the sound box is stuffed
full of anything, no music.
If the brain and the belly are burning clean with fasting
every moment a new song comes out of the fire.
The fog clears, and new energy makes you run up the steps
in front of you.
Be emptier and cry like reed instruments cry. Emptier, write
secrets with the reed pen.
When you're full of food and drink, Satan sits where your
spirit should, an ugly metal statue in place of the Kaaba.
When you fast, good habits gather like friends who want
to help.
Fasting is Solomon's ring. Don't give it to some illusion and
lose your power, but even if you have, if you've lost all will
and control, they come back when you fast, like soldiers

appearing out of the ground, pennants flying above them.
A table descends to your tents, Jesus's table.
Except to see it, when you fast, this table spread with other
food, better than the broth of cabbages."
Rumi (as translated by Coleman Barks, 1997)

FASTING TODAY

Celebrities are usually the first to focus attention on any technique that involves the body beautiful, and fasting is no exception. So, as part of my research for this book, I went in search of some of the world's most famous celebrity personal trainers to ask them if they use fasting with their clients.

The most logical place to start was to think of whose body I most admire. Easy – my ultimate body icon is Gwen Stefani. She's honest about the fact that her incredible physique is down to hard work and she's a real inspiration, especially for women who've had children – a mother of two, and yet look at her abs... Respect! I finally tracked down her personal trainer, Mike Heatlie. He has an impressive CV to go with an even more impressive body. He holds three degrees, including two Masters – in Medicine & Science in Sport and Exercise, and in Strength and Conditioning. Here's what he had to say:

> *"The vast majority of celebrities such as Gwen Stefani work*
> *their ass off to get in that type of condition. Gwen is the most*
> *hard-working client I've ever trained, and the results show it.*
> *If people saw the work she puts in to look as good as she does*
> *then people may say, 'well that's not for me, that's too much*

hard work'. Other celebrities such as Daniel Craig, Hugh Jackman and Hilary Swank all developed their physiques through sheer hard work. Of course they have Personal Trainers to help them but they have to put the work in themselves and diet properly.

I've used intermittent fasting on many occasions – notably when people need to lose those last 2–4.5kg [5–10lb], or in order to stimulate stubborn fat loss. I have one client who fasts every Wednesday, just drinks water, green tea, some amino acids, and that's it, and that works very well for her. There are many protocols for fasting and each individual can use the one that works best for them. As with all diets though, the protocol needs to be sustainable so it can be implemented into a lifestyle."

If you still believe that fasting is just another passing diet fad – here today, gone tomorrow – think again. As I mentioned in the Introduction, I predict that fasting will not only become the next big global health trend but that it's here to stay. From a professional point of view, a technique that gets results without compromising health, that helps restore a sense of calm in the mind, and that costs nothing to do, kind of has it all.

CHAPTER 2

EAT, FAST AND LOSE WEIGHT

THE TRUTH ABOUT FAT AND WEIGHT LOSS

These days, in countries where there's an abundance of food, we've become used to constant grazing – rarely sitting down for meals and simply picking at high-caloric, high-fat and high-sugar foods all day long. **We've forgotten what it feels like to be really physically hungry.**

The unfortunate truth is that many of us are *designed* to get fat. It all comes down to evolution. Back in the dim and distant past, when food shortages were common, people who had substantial fat "in storage" were more likely to survive.

Research carried out in the last century proved that extended periods of starvation are much less dangerous for people who have high levels of body fat – in fact, the heavier you are, the more likely it is that fasting will lead to substantial fat loss with muscle being spared. In contrast, the slimmer you are (and your ancestors were), the more likely it is that you'll break down muscle through extreme dieting.

People often blame their genes for a "slow metabolism" or "big bones", but it turns out things are more complicated than that. The genetic factors that helped your ancestors lay down fat stores seem to relate to a complex range of factors rather than simply affecting your metabolic rate. For example, there are subtle differences in appetite, or in the tendency to fidget.

TYPES OF FAT CELLS

Abdominal fat (sometimes called visceral fat) is found deep in your body surrounding your internal organs, whereas subcutaneous fat lies just below the surface of your skin – the stuff you can pinch with your fingers. You may think that being a little heavy around your middle isn't *such* a bad thing, but unfortunately recent research shows that **excess fat in this area – rather than on your thighs or bottom – increases your risk of diabetes, heart disease, *stroke*, high blood pressure and even certain cancers.** Scientists have found that abdominal fat is more biologically active than other fat cells in the body, meaning it produces more hormones and other biochemicals that can have a profound effect on your health. For example, abdominal fat produces immune system chemicals called *cytokines*, which have been shown to increase your risk of cardiovascular disease by promoting *insulin* resistance and low-level inflammation.

WHY SOME PEOPLE ARE NATURALLY SLIM

Emerging research suggests that naturally slim people have genetic advantages that make it easier for them to *avoid* weight gain. **They're not blessed with faster metabolisms, but tend to be able to regulate their appetite and burn off excess calories without even noticing it.**

TO THEM, FOOD IS JUST FOOD

Naturally slim people enjoy food, but they don't have a strong emotional connection to it. Foods aren't "good" or "bad", they're just food. Therefore, slim types don't feel guilty when they tuck into a slice of cake or have a few chips with their dinner.

THEY CAN STOP AFTER JUST ONE BITE

When our naturally slim friends eat indulgent foods, they can stop after just a little, rather than polishing off the plate. Many of us are familiar with that feeling of having broken the diet rules:

> *"That's today ruined… I may as well finish the whole cake and start again tomorrow."*

Slim people don't get that "all or nothing" feeling that's typical in seasoned dieters.

THEY RECOGNIZE THE DIFFERENCE BETWEEN HUNGER AND APPETITE

The mechanisms controlling our appetites are complex. Research suggests that naturally slim people may be more resistant to appetite signals that aren't linked to physiological hunger. What this means is, **they eat when their body needs nourishment, not when their brain is trying to trick them into believing they're hungry.** In contrast, those of us with a genetic tendency to gain weight can feel *physically* hungry when tempted by food, even if our bodies don't need the calories.

THEY BURN IT OFF

There's a theory that our body weight has a "set point" (a natural weight at which it tries to maintain itself). **When a naturally slim person overeats, they tend to compensate by moving around more, without even thinking about it.** So, as well as a few more gym sessions, they may fidget, get stuck into cleaning the house, or walk rather than taking the car. But for the majority of us, overeating is followed by a few hours relaxing on the sofa!

THEY GET ENOUGH SLEEP

In studies where people have been limited to four hours' sleep a night for several days, changes in appetite *hormones* have been observed, and the appetite for sweets, salty snacks, fatty and starchy foods seems to increase. Through sleeping longer, our naturally slim friends may find that they're less tempted to snack. There are more than 65 published research papers that have linked sleeping for fewer than six hours a night with increased weight. When researchers at the University of Warwick analyzed all the evidence on the relationship between sleep and obesity, they found that **adults who slept for fewer than five hours a night were one-and-a-half times more likely to be obese!**

OTHER FACTORS INFLUENCING WEIGHT

Ultimately, weight gain comes down to the fact that we're **eating more calories than we're burning off**, and over time this has led to many of us gradually getting fatter. But tackling the issue is about more than simply cutting calories. **The quality of what we eat is important too.** The types of food that are so readily available to us – those muffins and sugary drinks – tend to be packed with sugar or refined *carbohydrates* (*carbs*) and it's very easy to eat them and not notice when we're full. Instead, try replacing those "empty" calories with nutrient-rich, lean proteins, leafy green vegetables and even healthy fats from nuts and oily fish. I promise you, these will make you feel full and you'll be much less tempted to overeat.

It's also important to detect underlying problems or habits that can be causing or contributing to a weight problem. For example, **stress, emotional eating** or **chemical calories** may have been the tipping point for your body. Unhealthy eating can mean that you're not getting enough of the vitamins, minerals and essential fats that your body needs to function well. What's more, **many "fad" diets aren't nutritionally balanced**, so they starve the body of the vital nutrients your body needs.

On a basic level, these problems can make it very hard for you to stick to a diet. Likewise, **"crash" diets tend to drastically restrict your body's intake of calories**. If your body isn't getting the nutrients it needs, the result can be irritability, depression and even lowered brain function, all of which inevitably affect your **motivation to continue with the diet. And when you come off the diet, you quickly return to your previous weight and may end up gaining even more weight.** This is because, when you lose weight, your metabolic rate naturally dips – more about this shortly.

STRESS AND WEIGHT GAIN

The link between stress and weight gain begins with tiny glands called *adrenals*. Their basic task is to rush all your body's resources into "fight or flight" mode by increasing production of adrenaline and other hormones – you may recognize this feeling with an increased heart rate, and your blood pressure may be raised.

Unlike our ancestors, who weren't distracted by mobile phones, deadlines, emails and the multi-tasking challenges of modern life, today we live under constant stress. Instead of occasional, acute demands followed by rest, we're constantly over-worked, under-nourished, exposed to environmental toxins, and plagued by worries... with no let-up.

Every challenge to the mind and body creates a demand on the adrenal glands. The result is a state of constant high alert and high levels of the hormone *cortisol* in the body, leading to a huge number of health problems, such as a tendency to hold on to stubborn belly fat. The other main side-effects of stress and adrenal overload are digestive problems, rapid ageing, lowered immunity and skin problems.

Sometimes it's less about the stress in our lives and more about the stress we place on ourselves with what we eat and drink. Take caffeine, for example. We're all familiar with the "buzz" that caffeine can give. Many products are marketed solely on the basis of this false energy kick, but that lively feeling is actually the sensation of adrenaline being pumped around the body as a result of the caffeine hit. The adrenal glands tire of constant stimulation and when the inevitable adrenal fatigue kicks in, it leads to a slowdown in the conversion of stored fats (and proteins and carbohydrates) into energy. We experience this failure in the energy chain as a craving for further stimulants in the form of more caffeine from another cup of tea, coffee, cola drink or caffeinated beverage. The last piece of the picture with caffeine is what usually comes with it. Remember that **an average coffee these days contains a sizeable portion of milk, sugar or syrup** and then there's the ubiquitous temptation of a muffin or pastry accompaniment!

INSULIN RESISTANCE AND THE EFFECTS OF ALCOHOL

When the body is overloaded with carbs (which are extremely commonplace in the average Western diet), it has to respond by making more insulin. Carbs are broken down into molecules of the sugar *glucose*, and insulin is the hormonal "key" that unlocks the cells to allow the glucose in. Over a period of time, excess insulin affects the cells by making them less sensitive to taking sugars into the cell and creating energy. This in turn prevents the cells from burning fat. The good news is that **fasting may improve how your body handles sugar and help your body burn fat instead of storing it.**

As far as your body's concerned, alcohol is chemically similar to sugar, so **drinking any form of alcohol will set off the same insulin resistance seesaw that can promote weight gain.** And that's before you even begin to **consider the calorie content of the drink itself,** which is likely to be very high and devoid of any nutritional benefit – so-called "empty calories". What's more, **alcohol acts as a potent appetite booster,** so more alcohol equals more food consumed!

There's yet another reason behind alcohol's "beer belly" effect. **Alcohol reduces the amount of fat your body burns for energy, while preventing the absorption of many of the essential nutrients needed for successful weight loss,** particularly the B vitamins and vitamin C. In one study published in the *American Journal of Clinical Nutrition*, eight men were given two glasses of vodka with diet lemonade, each containing just under 90 calories. For several hours after drinking the vodka, the amount of fat the men burned dropped by a massive 73 percent. Because your body uses more than one source of fuel, if alcohol is consumed then this alcohol "energy" will be used instead of fat – not good news for the waistline!

EMOTIONAL EATING

As we all know, **a lot of eating is emotionally driven.** Many people with weight problems fear feeling hungry. Furthermore, reaching for the sugar-fix from food or from alcohol is what helps free us, temporarily, from whatever uncomfortable emotion we might be feeling. Of course, sometimes an eating problem masks an underlying psychological problem or challenge. In such cases, expert advice, counselling or psychotherapy or psychology can really help.

Even when eating is free from emotional factors, the fact is, the longer you spend on a diet (whether for health or for weight loss), the less strict you become and the more likely it is that calories will sneak in without you noticing – a bite of this here, a nibble of that there. Fasting shakes up this model of eating altogether. Having a large section of the day when food simply isn't allowed to pass your lips prevents random snacking, and might also alert you to how often you do this normally. **If you'd describe yourself as someone with limited self-control, fasting is an easier option than almost any other diet out there** as you don't have to count every calorie or become a slave to food group fads – the only thing you really need to do is watch the clock.

"CHEMICAL CALORIES"

It's thought that **chemicals in the environment have a blocking effect on the hormones that control weight loss.** When the brain is affected by these toxins, hormone signalling can be impaired. Reducing chemicals in our homes, foods and drinks is important when looking at the overall picture of weight loss and health. As you'll discover in the "Nutritional Rules for Fasting" chapter, one of my nutrition rules as part of any fasting programme is to eat real food rather than fake food. If you can't pronounce what it says on the label, you probably shouldn't be eating it!

THYROID PROBLEMS

An underactive thyroid can cause weight gain, too. Symptoms include fatigue, cold, hormonal problems, depression and low libido as well as unexplained weight gain. The challenge is sometimes that the problem is sub-clinical, in other words, your test from the doctor may come back negative but you still have the symptoms. This can be frustrating for the sufferer as it sometimes means a re-visit in six months to a year to see if the symptoms register as qualifying for medical intervention.

A nutritious diet designed with thyroid health in mind can help. For the thyroid to work optimally, it needs nutrients such as iodine, manganese, vitamin C, methionine, magnesium, selenium, zinc, and the *amino acids* cysteine and L-tyrosine. These are all found in healthy foods such as fruit, vegetables, nuts, seeds and meat.

WHAT YOU SHOULD WEIGH

Before you embark on a fasting programme for weight loss, let me help you establish what you should weigh. For many people, women in particular, the figure we think of as "ideal" is far removed from what is realistic, or even healthy. I could go on and blame the media or the fashion industry. We all know *that* argument and, yes, it's partly true.

Ironically, where I learned about fasting in India, the thought of using fasting to get slim would be abhorrent, as being skinny is associated with poverty and lower social castes. Fasting should never be used to strive for a body that's slimmer than is healthy – the size zero craze being a case in point. **The less body fat you have to lose, the more you need to ensure that fasting is not over-done since weight loss is a guaranteed side-effect.**

BODY MASS INDEX (BMI)

Healthy weight ranges are especially useful if you're already light for your frame – you've probably heard of BMI, which gives an indication of how healthy your current weight is in proportion to your height. The formula for calculating BMI is:

BMI = weight (kg) ÷ height (m)^2
(in other words, your weight in kilograms divided by your height in metres squared).

If maths isn't your strong point, you can find out your BMI using an online calculator.

A healthy BMI is between 18.5 and 24.9. Although many celebrities have a BMI below 18.5, this simply isn't healthy. Some studies suggest that the ideal BMI is 23 for men and 21 for women – particularly if it's a long and healthy life you're after.

However, if your BMI is, say, 25 you won't become magically healthier by losing 450g (1lb) and dieting down to a BMI of 24.9. In fact, it's perfectly possible for someone with a BMI of 27 to be much healthier than someone with a BMI of 23. That's because **BMI doesn't take your body fat, waist circumference, eating habits or lifestyle into account**. An example of this could be a professional rugby player who's heavier than average simply because he or she is very muscular. There's nothing unhealthy about having lots of muscle, but the BMI scale might say he or she is overweight or even obese. In contrast, a chain-smoker who lives on diet drinks and never exercises can have a so-called "healthy" BMI. Who do you think is healthier?

A BMI of 30 or above is considered "obese". A 2008 study by researchers at the Mayo Clinic in the USA, involving over 13,000 people, found that 20.8 percent of men and 30.7 percent of women were obese according to the BMI scale. But when they used the World Health Organization gold standard definition of obesity – measuring body fat percentage – 50 percent of the men and 62.1 percent of the women were classified as obese. (In other words, you can have a healthy BMI and an unhealthy level of body fat.) What this means is that the athlete who's unfairly classed as "obese" is the exception rather than the rule. Unless you're an avid weight-lifter or sportsperson, or you have an extremely physical job, the BMI scale isn't likely to tell you that you need to lose weight if you don't. If your BMI is well over 25, don't worry. Medical experts agree that losing 5–10 percent of your starting weight is a sensible and realistic initial goal that will have lasting health benefits.

Therefore, when it comes to the BMI scale, **it *is* worth calculating your BMI before deciding on a weight loss goal, especially if you only have a little weight to lose, but it definitely shouldn't be the only thing you think about.**

BODY FAT PERCENTAGE

What's great about monitoring your body fat percentage is that it gives you a better understanding of what's going on inside your body as you lose weight. Sustainable weight loss is best achieved through a combination of good nutrition and an active lifestyle. The thing is, **when you start exercising more, you often gain muscle mass.**

It can be demotivating to step onto the scales and see that your overall weight hasn't changed in spite of all your hard work. But because muscle is more dense than fat, you can look slimmer and achieve health benefits without actually losing weight. To track changes in your body fat, you need to invest in **body composition scales** which enable you to track your progress by measuring changes in your muscle mass, body fat and hydration. Gyms often have high-quality versions of these scales if you don't want to buy your own.

Body composition scales are also helpful because if you notice that your muscle mass is decreasing as rapidly as your body fat, this suggests that you've cut your energy intake too dramatically. **For most people, it's realistic to lose 450–900g (1–2lb) of body fat per week.** If you're losing much more than this, the chances are you're eating into your muscle mass. Body composition scales can alert you to this before you've risked damaging your health.

In women, it's normal for hydration levels to fluctuate along with the menstrual cycle. Again, measuring weight alone doesn't enable you to track these changes. By using the body composition scales at a similar time of day, and recording changes throughout the month, you can get a clearer understanding of the times you're gaining body fat, and when it's simply a matter of fluid retention.

Sophisticated body composition monitors also enable you to track abdominal fat. Remember, not all fat is created equal, and abdominal fat is concentrated around your vital organs, posing the biggest health risk. **You can be a "healthy" weight, and have high levels of abdominal fat** – being aware of this can give you the motivation you need to address your eating habits and activity level.

The scales use a weak electric current to differentiate between fat, muscle, fluid and bone – we won't go into too much detail here as different brands have different features. As a guide, if you're an ordinary adult, and not an athlete or aspiring fitness model, you should be aiming for the following body fat percentages:

AGE	MALE	FEMALE
20–39	8–20%	21–33%
40–59	11–22%	23–34%
60+	13–25%	24–36%

WAIST CIRCUMFERENCE AND WAIST-TO-HIP RATIO

One of the most useful basic measurements is the waist-to-hip ratio (WHR). It all goes back to apples and pears. Not about eating them, although that would be a good start, but which one your body shape is most like. Your WHR will put you either in the "apple-shaped" category (with more weight around the waist) or "pear-shaped" (with more weight around the hips).

I like the WHR because it's fairer than BMI, which doesn't take varying body structures into account. Put it this way... a curvaceous "Marilyn Monroe type" with a nipped-in waist can have exactly the same WHR as a 50kg (8st), size-8 slip of a girl. If you're someone who's using fasting to get your body into supermodel shape, you'll be interested in the calculation below.

Actress and model Liz Hurley has a WHR of 0.7 – even her face is said to be perfectly proportioned. Scientists have gleefully spent hours locked away in dark cupboards sizing her up (okay, I made the last bit up, but the scientists are real). They have declared that she's *scientifically and statistically* proven to be nature's perfect woman. However, like most models, Liz has just lucked out genetically. A WHR of below 0.8 is ideal for women. For men, those with a WHR score of 0.9 or below tend to be healthier. The important thing is that if your WHR is higher than this, you should be working on your shape as much as on your weight.

CALCULATING YOUR WHR

Calculating your WHR is fairly simple. Get out a tape measure and measure the circumference of your hips at the widest part. You can do it in centimetres or inches. Next, measure the smaller circumference of your natural waist (usually just above the belly button). To determine the ratio, divide your waist measurement by your hip measurement.

Ideally, aim to keep your waist circumference below 94cm (37in) if you're a man and below 80cm (31in) if you're a woman. If your waist is larger than 102cm (40in) if you're a man or 88cm (35in) if you're a woman, this is putting you at increased risk of health conditions such as diabetes and heart disease. As you'll discover in the "Eat, Fast and Perform Better" chapter, **fasting is a great way** to reduce body fat and maintain lean muscle, which will help get your waist into a healthier shape.

WHY TRADITIONAL DIETING MAKES YOU HUNGRY

Going on a traditional diet without adequate energy intake for long periods of time can make your metabolic rate plummet and your appetite soar. Say you reduce your calories to below 1,000 a day for a number of weeks to fit into a party dress, the chances are you'll feel hungry and fed up much of the time, and as soon as the party starts, you'll dive head first into all the foods you've been avoiding, re-gaining that lost weight in no time! This, in a nutshell, sums up the seesaw of the diet industry.

The real trick is to keep your body feeling fuller for longer. I'm not talking about choosing one ready-meal over another, it's about understanding how to manage hunger so you naturally eat less most of the time. Please note, I don't say all of the time. Special events and over-indulging every now and then is good for the soul.

In tandem with a good diet overall, fasting can be used to retrain your hunger without the need for appetite suppressants or dodgy supplements. When you begin to fast you will feel hungry at your usual meal times. However, if you choose not to eat at that time, the peaks and troughs of hunger start to level out. All this happens without a decrease in metabolic rate. It doesn't take a genius to recognize that if you feel hungry less often, you'll eat less and therefore lose weight. There's a biological explanation for this. **Feelings of hunger and satiety (feeling full) are controlled by two main hormones** produced within the body, *ghrelin* (even the word sounds hungry) and *leptin*. This dynamic duo of hormones has a powerful effect on how much food you eat and how much of what you've consumed you "burn off".

GHRELIN

This hormone seems pretty straightforward. **When your stomach's empty, it sends out some ghrelin to tell an area of your brain, the *hypothalamus*, that you ought to be eating.** You then feel ravenous. But research published in the *American Journal of Physiology* suggests that ghrelin levels also rise in anticipation of eating – you get hungry partly because you're *expecting* a meal, not just because you have an empty stomach.

On a traditional diet, you get a peak of ghrelin before every meal – but because you don't eat as much as you'd really like to, you never feel fully satisfied. When you're fasting, your ghrelin levels still rise, but anecdotal evidence suggests that over time your body finds this sensation easier to get used to, probably because of the changes in your meal patterns. There's also a theory that a nutritionally poor diet (think additive-packed "diet" meals) sends ghrelin rocketing faster than a nutrient-dense plan like the ones I recommend (see pages 178–80).

LEPTIN

This hormone is a little more complicated. You'll sometimes hear leptin referred to as a "master regulator" of fat metabolism. There are even whole diet books devoted to it.

Leptin is made by the fat cells – put simply, the more fat you have, the more leptin is produced. Like ghrelin, it sends a signal to the hypothalamus, but with the opposite effect. **Leptin is supposed to maintain your body fat at a healthy level by telling you to stop eating when you start to gain too much fat.** We all know it doesn't really work like that in practice – if it did, no one would be overweight. So, what happens?

Well, leptin also increases when you overeat – especially stodgy, carbohydrate-rich meals. This is because its release is triggered by insulin, which responds to an increase in blood glucose after a meal. So, if you're constantly eating without a proper break, your leptin levels will always be high. At first this is good – it should signal to your brain that it's time to put down that muffin – but it can lead to a very dangerous vicious circle. The theory is that, over time, **too much leptin leads to the brain becoming resistant to its effects.** As your brain stops recognizing what leptin is trying to tell it, you end up feeling hungry all the time, and are never satisfied by even the biggest meal.

When you follow a traditional weight-loss diet the reduction in your body fat means that your leptin levels fall. Combine that with the rise in ghrelin and you'll understand why you feel driven to eat and eat. The "yo-yo" diet cycle begins. In fact, Australian researchers have found that leptin and ghrelin levels can be messed up for more than a year after you reach your target weight. Your body's doing everything it can to gain that fat back.

Compare this with intermittent fasting. Some studies suggest that leptin levels fall after 12–36 hours of fasting, but others show no evidence of a change within up to 24 hours. Even if fasting does send your leptin levels plummeting, they quickly go back to normal when you start to eat – especially if your meals are rich in carbohydrates. So, rather than having lower leptin all the time (like you do on a normal diet), **those days or meals when you eat "normally" during fast and feed cycles mean that your body gets a boost of leptin and feels more satisfied.**

WHY MOST DIETS FAIL

This probably isn't the first book about weight loss you've ever read. I often say I've been down the diet road myself so many times that I could be a tour guide. If you're asking yourself why fasting is going to be any different, here are the facts you need to know:

- "Yo-yo" dieting is the bane of many people's lives, but even if you've lost and gained weight countless times, recent research has shown that it's possible to lose weight safely without messing up your metabolism.

- Burning off more calories than you eat is the *only* way to lose weight – and the simple truth is that you *will* lose weight if you manage to keep the number of calories you eat below the amount you burn off... boring but true.

There are hundreds of different ways to create a calorie deficit – as evidenced by the huge diet book, diet shake, diet bar and "miracle" weight-loss supplement industry. But there are two main reasons why diets never tend to live up to their expectations, especially as you get closer to your goal weight:

1 **Traditional diets misrepresent the calories in/calories out equation.**
We've all heard that 450g (1lb) of fat is roughly equal to 3,500 calories, so the traditional calorie-counting approach is to cut calories by 500–1,000 per day in order to lose 450–900g (1–2lb) per week. The trouble is, as you get slimmer you become lighter and that actually reduces the amount of calories you burn at rest (your basal metabolic rate). **So, in traditional weight-loss plans, weight loss is initially rapid but tends to slow down over time, even if you maintain that original calorie deficit. This can be very demotivating.**

2 **It's sticking to your chosen approach that's often the hard part.**
   Even if you get your calories exactly right, how boring does
   counting every calorie get? Demotivation – either as a result of
   not seeing the numbers on the scales going down as quickly as
   they were, or boredom – can lead to lapses, which slow down the
   rate of weight loss even further. When you go back to your old
   eating habits – surprise, surprise – you'll gain all the weight back,
   and a little more, as a result of the natural dip in basal metabolic
   rate (calorie burn) caused by your initial weight loss.

HOW FASTING MAKES A DIFFERENCE

FASTING MAY BOOST METABOLIC RATE

You're probably thinking, "If I start starving myself, won't that
be worse for my metabolism?" First of all, fasting is not starving
yourself, and **don't worry that eating *less often* will damage your
metabolism**. Losing weight naturally slows your basal metabolic
rate (the amount of calories you burn at rest) in proportion to the
amount of weight you lose, no matter which method you use. This
is because your daily energy (calorie) needs are directly related to
your age, height, gender and weight, in particular your lean body
mass (muscle). It *doesn't* mean that eating more often will fire up
your metabolism.

You'll hear over and over again that after a night of sleep, your
metabolism has ground to a halt and you need to eat breakfast to stoke
your metabolic fire. **The idea that "breakfast boosts metabolism"
is simply not true** – it hasn't been backed up by research at all. The
breakfast myth is based on the "thermic effect of food". Around 10
percent of our calorie burn comes from the energy that we use to
digest, absorb and assimilate the nutrients in our meals. Roughly

speaking, if you eat a 350-calorie breakfast, you'll burn 35 calories in the process. But notice that you've eaten 315 extra calories to burn that 35. No matter what time of day you eat, you'll burn off around 10 percent of the calories in your food through the thermic effect of food. So, whether you eat your breakfast at 7am, 10am or never, if you eat roughly the same amount and types of food overall, its effect on your metabolism will be the same.

In fact, all the research on fasting seems to show that eating less often could actually boost your metabolic rate. In one British study conducted at the University of Nottingham, a two-day fast boosted participants' resting metabolic rate by 3.6 percent. In another study by the same research group, 29 healthy men and women fasted for three days. After 12–36 hours, there was a significant increase in basal metabolic rate, which returned to normal after 72 hours. The exact mechanisms for why this happens aren't clear.

FASTING INCREASES FAT BURN

What *is* clear is that **more of the calories you use for fuel during fasting come from your fat stores.** Scientists can estimate what proportion of your energy is coming from fats and carbohydrates by measuring the amount of oxygen inhaled and the amount of carbon dioxide exhaled in your breath. The higher the proportion of oxygen to carbon dioxide, the more fat you're burning. As part of the same Nottingham study, findings proved that the proportion of energy obtained from fat rose progressively over 12–72 hours, until almost all the energy being used was coming from stored fat. This is incredible news really!

We're so often told to "breakfast like a king, lunch like a prince and dine like a pauper" with a view to becoming healthy, wealthy and wise. This is usually explained by telling us that breakfast kick-starts the metabolism – but it turns out that **eating breakfast doesn't boost your fat-burning potential at all.** In a small study on breakfast-eaters – published in the *British Journal of Nutrition* – a 700-calorie breakfast *inhibited* the use of fat for fuel throughout the day. Put simply, when we eat carbohydrates, we use it for fuel, and this prevents our bodies tapping into our stubborn stored fat. **Constant grazing might be what's keeping fat locked away in your belly, bum or thighs – and fasting is one way to release it.**

FASTING MAINTAINS LEAN MUSCLE

The more muscle you have, the more calories you burn at rest. And before you say you don't want big muscles, another way to put that is: the less muscle you lose as you drop in weight, the less your basal metabolic rate falls as you move toward your goal weight. (Remember, your basal metabolic rate is the rate at which you burn calories, so it's really important in order to make staying in shape easier in the long term.) Besides, muscle takes up less room than fat. So, a person with good lean muscle mass will take a smaller dress size or use a narrower belt notch than someone who doesn't have it.

Fasting is better than plain old calorie restriction when it comes to maintaining lean body mass. This is largely because fasting **triggers the release of *growth hormone (GH)*, which encourages your body to look for other fuel sources instead of attacking its muscle stores.** This is thought to be a survival advantage – back when humans were hunter gatherers it wouldn't have made sense for our muscle mass to reduce when food was scarce – we needed strong legs and arms to hunt down our dinner!

In one study carried out by researchers at Intermountain Medical Center in the USA, participants were asked to fast for 24 hours.

During this time, GH levels rose by a whopping 1,300 percent in women and 2,000 percent in men.

Many other studies have investigated the effects of fasting on GH. Like other hormones, GH levels rise and fall throughout the day and night. They tend to be highest at the beginning of a good night's sleep, when our stomachs are empty but our bodies are hard at work repairing in preparation for a new day. Larger or more frequent bursts of GH are released when we continue to fast and also when we take part in vigorous exercise.

GH acts by sending a signal to our fat cells to release some of their contents into the bloodstream. This enables us to use more fat for fuel, instead of burning mainly carbohydrates for energy. **GH is also thought to maintain concentrations of another hormone, *insulin-like growth factor (IGF-1)*, which helps our muscles to build more protein.**

This is totally different to what happens when you simply cut calories without changing how often you eat. When you hear people saying you should eat little and often to maintain your blood glucose levels, what they're telling you to do, in actual fact, is to avoid this state. This is because whenever you top up your blood glucose levels through eating, your body releases insulin to compensate, and GH levels never get a boost when insulin is around.

It's important to note that more isn't necessarily better when it comes to GH – what's key is resetting the balance between GH release (which happens in the fasted state) and insulin release (which happens in the fed state, however small your meal) in order to stimulate fat loss without losing lean muscle. **You never need to fear growing giant muscles as a result of fasting** – GH is released in waves and goes back to normal levels quickly as soon as your body has released enough fat to burn.

As mentioned earlier, if you're already slim, it's especially important not to overdo it when fasting. Research published in the academic journal *Obesity Research* shows that within just two days of complete fasting, there's a dramatic increase in the use of muscle for fuel in people who are already a healthy weight. This is because they have less fat available to burn overall. **Perhaps the advice for people who are already svelte but who want to fast for health benefits is to fast little and often rather than to eat little and often.**

FASTING PATTERNS GIVE YOU ENERGY WHEN YOU NEED IT

Alongside maintaining your muscle mass to reduce the dip in your metabolic rate that happens as you lose weight, fasting may help with stubborn weight in other ways.

There's a theory that the reduction in calorie burn typically seen after following a calorie-restricted diet may be related more to changes in activity level than to basal metabolic rate. When you're only eating, say, 1,200 calories day after day, it may be difficult to maintain the energy levels and motivation to exercise. But following an intermittent fasting pattern means that you can concentrate your workouts around the times when you're eating. **More energy means a tougher workout – and more calorie burn overall.**

COMMON QUESTIONS AND ANSWERS

Q *Isn't "not eating" dangerous?*

A It's very important to establish that **fasting is not starvation**, which, of course, *is* dangerous. What I'm talking about is the health benefits of increasing the gaps between meals or eating less from time to time.

Some people who are fully signed up to the merry-go-round of traditional dieting will argue that not eating is likely to induce a low-blood-sugar or "hypo" episode. Feeling faint, clammy and unable to concentrate are typical symptoms, happily offset by a visit to the vending machine or, for the health-aware, a snack such as an oatcake or nuts and seeds. **I'm not suggesting that snacking should be outlawed** – most of the time, I'm more than happy to tuck right in. But fasting challenges the assertion that we can't survive, or even thrive, without five mini-meals a day.

I accept that challenging the blood-sugar story isn't going to win me any popularity prizes. However, the reality of what science is telling us today is that **there's no medical consensus on the concept of low blood sugar**. The vast majority of us are perfectly capable of regulating our blood glucose level and, although we may feel ravenous between meals, going without food for a few hours won't cause the blood glucose to plummet and, even if it does, our self-preserving mechanisms will kick into action long before we pass out. What this means is that insulin's counter-measure, glucagon, will kick in, releasing those locked-up glucose stores into the blood and bringing the glucose level back within its normal range.

A few words of warning, though... Diabetic "hypos" are a different thing altogether, of course, and can be very dangerous, but they are drug-induced. For people diagnosed as diabetic but who are not yet on insulin medication, fasting has proved promising. In a year-long study on intermittent fasting, the group who fasted every other day stayed off diabetes medication for significantly longer.

Q *Won't I feel light-headed and really hungry on a fast?*

A You might be worried that your blood sugar levels will dip too low between meals and that you'll feel faint and weak. But when you're not eating, other hormonal signals trigger your body to release *glucose* or make more. In one Swedish study by researchers at the Karolinska Institute, students who'd reported that they were sensitive to hypoglycaemia (low blood sugar) felt irritable and shaky during a 24-hour fast, but there was actually no difference in their blood sugar levels – it may all have been in their minds.

It's true that your brain requires about 500 calories a day to keep the grey matter ticking over effectively. The brain's preferred fuel is glucose, which your liver stores around 400 calories-worth of at a time. In a longer fast, the body is forced to increase its production of *ketone bodies*, which act as a glucose-substitute for your brain. But in the short term, **so long as you eat well before and after your fasting period, your body is perfectly able to produce enough glucose to keep your brain happy.**

Q *Hang on a minute… My trainer told me that six small meals will fire up my metabolism and stop me feeling peckish. Who's right?*

A This is one of those fitness and nutrition "truths" that has been repeated so many times, people are convinced that it's a fact. In one small study at the US National Institute on Aging, researchers found that people who ate only one meal a day did tend to feel hungrier than those who ate three. **But beyond eating three meals a day, meal frequency doesn't seem to make a difference to hunger or appetite**, so it comes down to what's actually easiest for you. A study published by the *International Journal of Obesity* showed that people who are overweight tend to snack *more* often.

The truth is, **you *will* feel hungry when fasting** – there's no getting away from that – **but rather than a constant unsatisfied feeling, your hunger will come in waves**. You'll start to recognize the difference between physical and psychological hunger. And you'll get to eat meals that are big enough to leave you feeling genuinely satisfied when you do eat.

Q *Surely after the fast is over, I'll be tempted to binge?*

A Dr Krista Varady, from the University of Illinois in Chicago, has been studying alternate-day fasting (ADF), a form of intermittent fasting, for several years. Her research studies put people on a strict calorie limit every other day. For women, this provides 400–500 calories a day and for men 500–600 calories a day, which is all eaten at lunchtime. On the alternate "feed day" participants can eat as much as they want, with no restrictions.

After a day of partial fasting, it turns out that people rarely gorge themselves on the feed day. Participants in the study ate, on average, around 110 percent of their energy requirements, which means that over the two days their calorie intake was similar to what it would be on a traditional diet.

That's why the outcomes on weight loss are similar – but **wouldn't you rather eat as much as you like every other day rather than constantly feel like you're "on a diet"?**

But watch out... a couple of recent studies by researchers at Cornell University in the USA and Imperial College, London, suggested that after a fast, people *are* more likely to reach for stodgy or fatty foods first, so make sure you follow the guidance in later chapters in order to ensure that all your nutritional bases are covered.

Q *Can fasting change my shape?*

A For many women, that last bit of surplus weight is carried around the hips and thighs and it simply won't shift. To solve this problem I suggest looking to the true body professionals.

According to noted intermittent-fasting expert Martin Berkhan, there's a good reason for this. All the cells in our body have "holes" in them known as receptors. To switch activity on and off in those cells, hormones or enzymes enter the receptors. **Fat cells contain two types of receptor – beta 2 receptors, which are good at triggering fat burning, and alpha 2 receptors, which aren't.** Guess which is mostly found in the fat stores of your lower body? Yes, our hips and thighs have nine times more alpha 2 receptors than beta.

Fasting is the only thing that alters alpha 2 receptor expression in adults – when we're fasting, the alpha 2 receptors are more likely to stay hidden. If you combine this with the fact that GH and *catecholamines* (hormones released by the adrenal glands) are particularly good at encouraging fat loss, then fasting is a way for your body to release the stubborn fat it retained while you were on traditional diets.

Q *What about belly fat?*

A All over the Internet you'll see promises that you can get rid of belly fat in a matter of days by taking supplements. We all know that this is simply not true. Stubborn fat around the middle is linked to a number of factors – including stress, alcohol, lack of exercise and a diet high in refined carbohydrates.

Every time you eat something sweet or a refined carbohydrate such as biscuits or white bread, your blood sugar levels rise quickly, causing your pancreas to release the fat-storing hormone, insulin. If you spend the day going from sugary snack to sugary snack, and especially if you wash everything down with a couple of glasses of wine, your body ends up storing more of the calories you eat and you end up with that dreaded "muffin top"!

Stress + refined carbohydrates + alcohol = a recipe for belly fat, especially if you're unlucky enough to be genetically predisposed to weight gain around the middle.

Q *How does fasting help torch belly fat?*

A To burn belly fat, free fatty acids must first be released from your fat cells (this is called *lipolysis*) and moved into your bloodstream, then transferred into the *mitochondria* of muscle or organ cells, to be burned (a process known as *beta-oxidation*).

Glucagon (another pancreatic hormone that has pretty much an equal and opposite effect to insulin) rises around four to five hours after eating, once all the digested nutrients from your last meal have been stored or used up. The purpose of glucagon is to maintain a steady supply of glucose to the brain and red blood cells, which it achieves by breaking down stored carbohydrates and leftover protein fragments in the liver. It also activates hormone-sensitive *lipase*, which triggers the release of fat from the fat cells, allowing other cells to be fuelled by fat as opposed to glucose.

When you're fasting, belly fat can be turned into energy to keep your organs working effectively and, for example, to provide power to the muscles that hold you upright, as well as fuelling muscle movement.

In contrast, when you're constantly grazing, your body doesn't need to release glucagon. Instead, the pancreas pumps out insulin, which also acts to maintain blood glucose levels within a narrow range. Insulin encourages the fat cells to keep their fat tightly locked up. Not only that, but any spare glucose that isn't required for energy and cannot be stored can actually be converted into fat.

Simply put, the body burns more fat in a fasted state, whereas, in the fed state, insulin causes fat to be taken up into the fat cells around your tummy (and elsewhere) for storage.

In one study, carried out at the Beltsville Human Nutrition Research Center in the USA, where weight loss wasn't even a planned outcome, cutting meals down to one per day compared to three per day (without restricting calorie intake), led to a 2kg (4lb 8oz) loss of body fat in eight weeks.

While no studies have been carried out specifically to investigate how fasting affects your waist circumference, it's been observed that people with high levels of belly fat tend to have lower levels of growth hormone. So in theory it makes sense that fasting is a better way to reduce belly fat than traditional dieting.

Q *What else can I do to help get rid of belly fat?*

A Endurance exercise selectively reduces abdominal fat and aids maintenance of lean body mass, so it's great to do in combination with intermittent fasting. Choose a fasting method that will enable you to take regular exercise – **gentle activity such as walking will help, but high-intensity training is even better.**

Also, a very small recent study, carried out at the University of Oklahoma in the USA, found that quality protein intake was inversely associated with belly fat, so make sure you **fuel up on lean proteins** (which your fasting plans are rich in), when you *are* eating.

Q *What about losing that last 4.5kg (10lb)?*

A This is often the hardest weight to shift. Not only that, it tends to creep back over a matter of weeks after you've finally reached your target weight. A familiar story is the strict diet we follow to get into beach-body shape in time for a holiday: in all the years I've helped people to lose weight, I've lost count of the number of times I've heard people telling me that all their hard work was undone by two weeks of sun, sea and sangria!

Remember that losing weight is all about creating a calorie deficit. Here, fasting is acting in two different ways. **First, fasting helps maintain calorie burn – so in theory you can eat more overall and still lose weight. Second, fasting might just be easier to stick to than a boring calorie-counting diet.** And when it comes to beach bodies, remember that old saying "a change is as good as a rest". If you're bored of the approach you've taken to weight loss up to now, a short blast of fasting can help you achieve your goal weight *without* damaging your metabolism.

This is backed up by research. **Most of the studies on intermittent fasting show that it can be just as effective for fat loss as traditional diets,** but the studies are all designed differently so it's difficult to say exactly which fasting approach will be the most effective for you. Scientific studies on intermittent fasting have shown varying results – from an average weight loss of a few kilos in the first few days, to 8 percent of body weight within eight weeks.

During the first few days of the fast you'll generally lose weight quickly, which can feel very motivating, especially if the scales have been stuck for a while.

One thing to note is that your weight *will* fluctuate. At first, you'll lose water (because stored glucose holds roughly four times its weight in water, and is quickly used up during a fast), and yesterday's food should make its way through your digestive tract. Alongside this, you'll lose some body fat. But the next day, you'll gain weight via the new intake of water and food. Don't worry! Over time, your average weight will fall. That's why it's important to **limit weighing yourself to once or twice a week**, and to be consistent in the time and day you use the scales.

WEIGHT-LOSS CASE STUDIES

In deciding to write this book, I was determined to make the science more real. Actions speak louder than words, and nothing gives more credence to the beneficial and gentle effects of fasting than hearing from people who've done it.

I'd used juice fasting with hundreds of people over the previous ten years and knew it could help kick-start weight loss as well as tackle troublesome health symptoms, but I was a relative newcomer to intermittent fasting. I'd seen the impressive before-and-after shots on fitness websites like *Lean Gains*, and read all the scientific studies, but I needed to know how intermittent fasting would work on ordinary men and women who were struggling to get rid of those last 4.5kg (10lb) or who wanted to shift stubborn fat around the middle.

Six members from my weight-loss website, who were at various stages of their weight-loss journeys, agreed to be my guinea pigs. The results were really impressive. In just six weeks, they lost an average of:

- 5.6kg (12lb 8oz)
- 7.4 percent of their body fat
- 5.8cm (2.3in) from their waist – that's a whole dress or trouser size!

Some of their stories appear below.

OVERCOMING A WEIGHT-LOSS PLATEAU

REAL-LIFE EXAMPLE
NAME: Karen McKay
AGE: 38
HEIGHT: 1.8m (5ft 3in)
WEIGHT BEFORE: 67.5kg (10st 10lb)
WEIGHT AFTER: 62.1kg (9st 12lb)
LOST: 5.4kg (12lb)

Self-confessed "huge eater" Karen had already lost over 6.3kg (1st) in two months by following my portion-controlled plans (based on three meals and two snacks a day). At the start of the trial, she weighed 67.5kg (10st 10lb) but was still 6.3kg (1st) away from her ultimate goal, and her weight had reached a plateau.

"I'd always half-heartedly been on a diet but when I couldn't get into my work trousers after Christmas I decided it was time for a totally different approach. I liked Amanda's really fresh approach to healthy eating. I was determined to stick to the plan, and very quickly I'd lost the first 10lb [4.5kg], although the weight losses were smaller after that."

Karen continued to follow my healthy eating menus, but switched from five small meals a day to a 16/8 fasting pattern, in which she fasted from 8pm in the evening until 12pm the next day. This meant skipping breakfast and her usual morning snack, then having an early lunch and a more substantial afternoon snack than usual. She slipped up a few times over the six weeks, even giving in to the temptation of some chocolate Easter eggs, but she still overcame the weight-loss plateau and lost a steady 900g (2lb) a week.

"For me this diet has been totally life changing. Before, it was all about white bread, eating on the hop and huge portions. I've had a couple of blips along the way but I've totally changed the way I eat. The most incredible thing is that I've even managed to get into a size 10! I couldn't even get into a size 14 after Christmas. I still can't quite believe it. But this is me now – I'm determined and, as long as the kids keep me running around after them the whole time, hopefully I can stay this way."

Karen noticed that her appetite tends to fluctuate alongside her monthly cycle. Look out for information on this in the "Me Tarzan, You Jane" chapter (see pages 120–30), which explains why fasting may work slightly differently for men and women. As a result, Karen continued following the 16/8 fasting pattern after the trial ended, but began eating breakfast every day during the final week of her cycle to help satisfy cravings.

Six months later, Karen is still maintaining her weight loss.

FITTING WEIGHT LOSS AROUND A BUSY WORK SCHEDULE

REAL-LIFE EXAMPLE
NAME: Juli Glasgow
AGE: 24
HEIGHT: 1.5m (5ft)
WEIGHT BEFORE: 76.5kg (12st 2lb)
WEIGHT AFTER: 70.2kg (11st 2lb)
LOST: 6.3kg (14lb)

Juli had only just signed up to my weight-loss site when I started looking for volunteers. She had an ambitious weight-loss goal – aiming to lose more than 19kg (3st) overall – and wanted a weight-loss plan that would fit her busy working life.

Juli followed a 5/2 fasting pattern, which meant that she ate a balanced menu five days a week, including three meals and up to two snacks. On the other two days, she was restricted to a small evening meal, averaging around 500 calories. This meant that she could structure her fasting pattern around the days when she'd be busiest at work – it's often easier to skip meals when you're busy, and it takes away the temptation to run for the vending machine rather than sit down to a proper meal. We also agreed that Juli could have one day off a week, usually at the weekend, when she didn't strictly follow my menu. It was this flexibility that most appealed to Juli:

> *"I find it so rewarding to have snacks off-plan on one day, and find it much easier to get back on plan 100 percent after. Everything is structured, and on a working day it's so easy to follow."*

Despite these planned "lapses" through weekend socializing, Juli also lost weight steadily and was a third of the way toward her ultimate goal by the end of the six weeks. Not only that, more of the weight went from around her tummy than her upper body. **Her waistline shrank by an amazing 7.6cm (3in) during the trial!**

LOSING WEIGHT WHEN EXERCISE IS IMPOSSIBLE

REAL-LIFE EXAMPLE
NAME: **Sinead O'Neill**
AGE: **40**
HEIGHT: **1.6m (5ft 4½in)**
WEIGHT BEFORE: **68.5kg (10st 13lb)**
WEIGHT AFTER: **63kg (10st)**
LOST: **5.85kg (13lb)**

Like Karen, Sinead had already lost almost 6.3kg (1st) when she began the trial. She was feeling very motivated to reach her goal weight – another 6.3kg (1st) away – in time for her 40th birthday, and was keen to avoid a weight-loss plateau. A fractured foot meant Sinead was unable to exercise, so the intermittent fasting plan appealed to her as an alternative way to accelerate weight loss.

"I found it really easy – I did six days of no breakfast, but incorporated the same number of calories into the rest of the day's food and it really worked. I got to my goal weight by my birthday and was delighted to get into a size 12 dress (my husband's reaction was incredible!) and I've also worn leggings again, which I never thought I would. The plan has given me incredible confidence and I have so much more energy now."

Sinead soon recovered from her broken foot, and started back at her exercise classes with a new-found confidence.

CHAPTER 3

EAT, FAST AND LIVE LONGER

THE HEALING POWER OF FASTING

What started as a personal experiment in an ashram in the Himalayas went on to become my number one method for treating age-related concerns, skin complaints, weight problems and digestive problems. Over the last decade I've seen my clients achieve amazing results with fasting. Getting to the optimum weight for your body frame is as much about health as it is about looking and feeling good. **Fasting improves health alongside helping to shift the pounds and, just as importantly, it can help heal somebody's relationship with food**, which is often at the heart of the struggle with weight.

I firmly believe that what I can achieve with a client during a week of fasting would take me months or possibly years with a conventional nutrition approach. In fact, I'll stick my neck out and say that fasting can and will change how we as a society view healing – if someone told you there was a pill that could reduce the risk of diabetes, cancer and heart disease and keep you looking and feeling young, you'd be tempted to take it, wouldn't you?

Unlike medication, **so long as you're sensible about it (see the "Fasting Safely" chapter), there are no harmful side-effects of fasting**. Contrast this with the side-effects of common prescription and over-the-counter drugs – even if the chance of side-effects is small, the risks are still real. One study published by the peer-reviewed *British Medical Journal* into the side-effects of statins (cholesterol-lowering drugs), confirmed cases of increased risk of muscle weakness, cataracts, acute kidney failure, and moderate or severe liver dysfunction. Of course, if disease has taken hold, the benefits of medication will often outweigh the risks. However, we need to be working toward a model of preventative action.

WHY WE NEED A NEW APPROACH

According to the World Health Organization, **2.8 million people die each year as a result of being overweight or obese.** We're all getting heavier, and in the past 30 years, obesity rates have almost doubled. Estimates of the *direct* National Health Service (NHS) costs of treating overweight, obesity and related morbidity in England alone have grown from £479.3 million a year in 1998 to £4.2 billion in 2007. The indirect annual cost to the economy, including lost productivity, is estimated at as much as £15.8 billion.

In 2008, two-thirds of all deaths worldwide were the result of non-communicable diseases – predominantly cardiovascular disease and cancer. **Eighty percent of all cardiovascular disease is thought to be caused by poor lifestyle choices, and some of the risk factors, such as high levels of fat and sugar in the blood and being overweight, can be improved through fasting.**

High blood sugar is also a risk factor for type-2 diabetes. The number of people with diabetes worldwide is rising at an alarming rate. In Britain, 1 in 20 people have already been diagnosed with diabetes, and 400 people are newly diagnosed every day. As there are no obvious signs and symptoms, it's been estimated that 850,000 Britons and 7 million Americans have diabetes and don't even know yet.

Of course, fasting isn't the only way to tackle these conditions – improving your diet generally, getting a bit more active, quitting smoking, drinking in moderation and limiting stress are all important – but fasting might just be the secret weapon you haven't yet discovered.

The great news is that fasting is going mainstream. Studies and research are beginning to prove what some people have known for a long time – that fasting not only prolongs life, but results in a marked degree of regeneration and rejuvenation. In fact, one of the amazing *proven* side-effects of fasting is that it helps to slow ageing at a cellular level. Yes, ditch the lotions and potions, there's a much more effective anti-ageing strategy that costs you nothing!

HOW FASTING PROMOTES HEALING

Nothing in the body, or mind, works in isolation, so it shouldn't come as a surprise to learn that fasting creates a healthy "ripple effect" of sorts.

The over-arching theory is that **fasting helps to de-stress the body**. When you fast you give your body a break and a chance to catch up on its inner "to-do" list. We all know how good it feels to have a well-earned holiday and return rested, rejuvenated and with a renewed *joie de vivre*. Well, fasting has a similar effect on your body.

Around 70 percent of your daily energy is spent maintaining internal functions, such as digestion and detoxification. If you're a busy, on-the-go person and don't give your body the best conditions to rest, digest and ultimately heal, ill-health will catch up with you sooner or later.

Have you ever had that sluggish feeling, much like a slow hangover that's really difficult to shake off? Just as your home or office can become dusty and dirty, so your body can become clogged up with toxins and waste matter from the environment around you (more about this later in the chapter). **When your body is clean and strong, it's able to eliminate toxins efficiently**, but when it becomes overloaded it can become sluggish, overweight (or underweight in some instances) and more susceptible to disease. The result is that "toxic signals", such as aches and pains, irritable bowel, skin complaints, mood swings and fatigue, start to kick in. If these signals are ignored, they allow longer-term chronic health problems to take hold.

Cue fasting. Thousands of studies or observations of both man and animals have established the fact that when the body goes without food, the tissues are called upon in an inverse order of their importance to the organism. What this means is that **when you fast, fat is the first tissue to go**. And, contrary to expectations, instead of food deprivation causing a debilitating loss of nutrients, in short-term fasts the body retains the majority of these.

When you fast, the body is also given the time to identify and get rid of damaged or defective parts. This process is called autophagy. The term was coined by a biochemist in the 1960s and means "self-eating", which sounds like something from a zombie B-movie, so it's better to think of it as a spring clean for your body. For example, when mitochondria (the cellular generators responsible for energy output) progressively lose function and become damaged due to ill-health and bad diet, this intensifies the rate of cellular ageing and the onset of death. Mitochondrial dysfunction has been linked to a variety of illnesses including diabetes, heart disorders and neurological problems. **Autophagy enables the cells to get rid**

of the dysfunctional mitochondria, allowing them to be replaced by more "energy efficient" new ones. It also helps the body to fight infections and recover from injuries.

This makes even more sense when you consider that at any one time only about half of your cells are at the peak of development, vitality and working condition. A quarter of them are usually in the process of development and growth and the other quarter are in the process of dying and being replaced. **During a fast the process of elimination of the dead and dying cells is speeded up and the building of new cells is accelerated and stimulated.** At the same time, the toxic waste products that interfere with the nourishment of the cells are effectively eliminated and the normal metabolic rate and cell oxygenation are restored.

Fasting is now considered an acceptable treatment or approach for promoting longevity, improving insulin response, reducing inflammation, boosting cardiovascular health and even for supporting cancer treatment. Fasting may deliver health benefits and more, without many of the unpleasant side-effects produced by other treatments, and, again, without an extortionate price tag.

FASTING AND ANTI-AGEING

Ageing is inevitable. Everything that keeps us alive from one day to the next can be called your metabolism, and running your body has side-effects. Those side-effects accumulate and eventually will cause problems. Welcome to the reality of ageing... But reality is ever changing and there's good reason to be optimistic. Like looking for the proverbial pot of gold, we seekers of health are all out there, trying to find the elixir of youth.

You're as young or as old as your smallest vital links – your cells. Ageing begins when your normal process of cell regeneration and rebuilding slows down. **At a cellular level, the hormone insulin-like growth factor (IGF-1) has both positive and negative effects.** Like insulin, it's anabolic, meaning that, in effect, it tells our cells to grow and multiply. If IGF-1 is kept high, our cells constantly divide and multiply, which is good if we're trying to build big muscles and not so good if those cells become damaged and cancerous. High levels of IGF-1 have been linked to prostate cancer and post-menopausal breast cancer. When IGF-1 levels drop, the body slows production of new cells and starts repairing old ones, and *DNA* damage is more likely to be permanent.

What does all this mean for adding years to our life? Headed by gerontologist Valter Longo, researchers at the University of Southern California in the USA have focused for the last decade on the effect of calorie restriction on the functioning of cells. When Longo and his researchers began exploring the links between food intake and longevity, **research on mice found that restricting calories extended lifespan by up to 40 percent.** Genetically engineering the mice to have low levels of IGF-1 did the same thing.

Other research on our monkey cousins has shown that, in most cases, both calorie restriction and intermittent fasting helps them to live longer. In fact, it appears that the more they fast and the less they eat, the longer they live. Sounds crazy, doesn't it? After all, we're much more used to hearing ourselves say we're going to "starve to death" or that we'll "waste away" if we go a few hours without a decent meal.

Lower levels of IGF-1 work for people too. During the Great Depression there were food shortages and drought, yet life expectancy actually rose by six years from 1929 to 1933. Intrepid scientists have also found populations of people where the rules of ageing don't apply. Settlers in a remote region of Ecuador who have low levels of IGF-1 seem to be "immune" to diabetes and cancer, despite their very unhealthy lifestyle. However, it's not something that can be bottled, or not yet anyway. The Ecuadorians who have demonstrated this mind-boggling immunity have a pre-existing condition called *Laron Syndrome* (this comes with growth problems, so it isn't the magic answer). In fact, the only way you can naturally reduce levels of IGF-1 these days is by choosing to fast, rather than waiting for life to force it upon you. The benefits come quickly – within just 24 hours of fasting, IGF-1 falls.

BLOOD SUGAR CONTROL

The truth is that **with a typical Western diet it's easy to be hungry all the time**. Many of you will smile ruefully at the feeling. Think about it – the "low-fat" foods that fly off the shelves every diet season are full of sugar and artificial sweeteners which are addictive and increase cravings for more of the same.

The idea of eating little and often, which is promoted by so many diet plans, is about preventing your body from releasing too much insulin at once and only giving it the nutrients that it can immediately put to use. But in order to burn off body fat, your insulin levels need to be low. So, if you eat little and often, your body will always be releasing a little insulin. **If you're someone who eats all the time, you may have chronically high insulin levels.** Insulin provides the signal to your body to store energy from your food so that it can be accessed later. It basically acts by unlocking cells and allowing individual molecules of glucose to enter. It also tells the cells to make more protein and fat and to keep the existing fat locked away inside. This is all designed at keeping the levels of blood sugar within a tightly controlled range.

Any sugar that isn't immediately required for energy has to be stored in the muscles or liver. **High levels of insulin in the body can increase the risk of insulin resistance** (those locks get "broken" and start having difficulties recognizing the "key"). **Over time, insulin resistance increases the risk of diabetes and has also been linked to cardiovascular disease, cancer and other inflammatory health conditions.**

Most studies on fasting suggest that it has a beneficial effect on blood glucose control. Increasing the gaps between meals through fasting means that you get a spike in insulin after eating, then a longer period of time where insulin isn't involved at all. The idea is that this not only encourages your body to burn fat, it also helps to maintain its natural sensitivity to insulin.

FASTING AND INFLAMMATION

Inflammation is the body's normal response to injury, and is aimed at removing whatever's causing the injury and kick-starting the healing process. Too much inflammation can obviously be dangerous, as is the case in inflammatory conditions such as arthritis, atherosclerosis and even eczema. If you or someone you know has a condition that ends in "-itis", it's linked to inflammation.

High levels of body fat are associated with increases in inflammatory markers such as Interleukin-6 (*IL-6*), Tumour Necrosis Factor-alpha (*TNFa*) and C-Reactive Protein (*CRP*). **Studies on several different fasting formats show that these inflammatory markers tend to reduce during periods of fasting.** This is the case during Ramadan (when Muslims practise a daily fast of 12–18 hours throughout the ninth month of the Islamic calendar), and also for a single daily meal versus three meals a day, and for alternate-day fasts. Intermittent fasting has been specifically shown to reduce the symptoms of asthma, another condition in which inflammation plays a key role.

REAL-LIFE EXAMPLE
NAME: **Lorraine Elkins**

Lorraine's health took a dramatic turn for the worse in the spring of 2009. Within a few months, symptoms of rheumatoid arthritis (RA), a debilitating autoimmune condition, turned her from a high-flyer in banking to someone who could barely walk. RA is known as a particularly difficult condition to treat, and the normal method often has onerous side-effects. There is no proven medical cure as yet. Lorraine describes how she felt:

> *"It was a really difficult time. I had no energy to do anything. It was even difficult to sleep when the pain was at its worst. I couldn't even manage to hang my washing out or walk around a local shop without having to stop and rest. I was unrecognizable to myself and was incredibly down about it all. I remembered Amanda from her TV show, "The Spa of Embarrassing Illnesses", and decided to get in contact – although if I'm perfectly honest, I didn't hold out much hope as my symptoms were just so awful."*

Lorraine visited me initially for a clinic consultation. As she described her symptoms, my heart went out to her. I knew that small changes wouldn't work – the effect of nutrition can often be subtle and long term. So, I recommended the only course of treatment that I believed could help – a juice-fasting programme which was starting on a retreat the following week.

Lorraine recalls:

> *"I checked into Amanda's retreat feeling like a lump of cement. I was exhausted, miserable and sore. I didn't really believe it would work but was willing to try anything. The first two days were really hard. Bizarrely, on the second night I had the strangest dreams I can remember of my adult life. They are still vivid even now. When I woke up, I remember feeling like something had changed. It was like energy dust had been sprinkled over me. I had forgotten what this felt like. I'm a black-and-white, traditional person, yet I'm not ashamed to say I cried. It was a glimmer of how I used to be.*
>
> *"I called my husband and he said, 'You're back'. It was so profound, even my voice sounded like me again. I went on from there and gained confidence. I believed the fasting programme worked with the drugs, not against them. When I went back for my weekly blood test the results were amazing! The overall measure of inflammation had dropped to near-normal levels and my immune system marker (which had been three times the healthy level) was back in the normal range."*

Luckily, the doctors have been incredibly supportive. Lorraine's medical team even asked her to tell their other patients about her experience. They acknowledge that this kind of approach is outside the realm of what would normally be prescribed on the NHS, but the results have been so undeniably positive that they fully support the approach.

Now, several years on, Lorraine's RA is really well managed – to the extent that her condition is no longer a day-to-day concern. She calls the juice-fasting programme "The Big Boys" – the tools that can be deployed if she ever goes off track. She believes that the fasting approach helps her body to create an internal "shift" that then allows the more traditional treatment approach to work much more effectively. It's the perfect example of a collaborative approach.

KEEPING THE HEART AND CIRCULATION HEALTHY

Inflammation is involved in cardiovascular disease, in concert with high levels of "bad" fats in the blood. Most studies on fasting show that it reduces *triglyceride* levels and improves the ratio of triglycerides to "good" *cholesterol* (that is, *high-density lipoprotein* [*HDL*] – the transport protein that helps remove excess cholesterol from the bloodstream). In animal studies, resistance to what is known as "ischaemic injury" – the type of artery damage that's associated with the build-up of plaques and hardening of the arteries – has been seen.

All in all, although the findings are far from clear and lots more research is needed, **fasting seems to give the body an internal tune-up and to increase resistance to age-related illnesses.**

Going back to those scary statistics from the beginning of this chapter – **cardiovascular disease is the leading cause of death worldwide** and something that affects us all. In Britain, NHS statistics show that in England in 2007, people aged over 60 were prescribed an average of 42.4 prescription items each. Each time you receive a prescription for an individual drug from your doctor, it counts as one prescription item. That's a whole lot of drugs! Unsurprisingly, medication that treats cardiovascular disease and its risk factors is the most commonly prescribed. I often meet people who want to change their eating habits, not just because they'd like to look and feel better, but because they're shocked by the amount of medication that their own parents are on. As fasting becomes more popular, people are becoming attracted to it as a lifestyle choice that might help their heart and circulatory system stay healthy for longer.

REAL-LIFE EXAMPLE
NAME: Claire Skinner

After Claire's 72-year-old mother suffered a deep vein thrombosis (DVT) on a flight to Hong Kong, electrocardiogram results showed that she had suffered a heart attack about 20 years previously. As a result her left ventricle was barely pumping. The cardiologist warned that Claire and her brother had at least a 10 percent chance of having heart problems.

On hearing this and having watched a TV documentary about the benefits of fasting, Claire felt she owed it to herself to at least give fasting a try.

> *"Fasting wasn't as difficult as I expected it to be and I felt great. Within a few weeks of starting, I requested via my GP to have a heart health screen because of my mother's findings. I had an electrocardiogram (ECG) and blood tests. My doctor was extremely pleased with the results, stating that whatever I was doing, I should continue with it! In my family there's significant history of heart disease, stroke, cancer and diabetes, so I'm more than willing to do (virtually) anything to decrease my chances of developing these diseases. I don't weigh myself – I prefer to go on how I feel and how my clothes fit. In the first week, I lost 6cm [2½in] and after eight weeks*

I'd lost 6cm [2½in] from my chest and hips, and 5cm [2in] from my waist – a great bonus for doing something that's health motivated."

FASTING AND CANCER

Fasting is considered to be an alternative or complementary treatment for cancer in certain sectors of complementary medicine, and has been popularized by a naturopathic doctor called Max Gerson. However, **my focus is not on fasting as a stand-alone treatment** but rather on exciting evidence about fasting in cancer prevention and the encouraging results from trials involving fasting during cancer treatment, particularly chemotherapy.

There's evidence that intermittent fasting, and calorie restriction more generally, fights the growth and spread of cancer cells in animals. Often when we read about research on animals, it seems so compelling that we want to see if the same thing will work for us. However, research is so much less likely to be done on humans as, rightly or wrongly, ethics committees are often reluctant to approve the same types of study that are done on animals. As discussed above, in experiments on laboratory animals, diets with 25 percent fewer calories have shown a positive link with longer, healthier life spans. **So far there's little empirical study evidence to show the same effect in humans, yet anecdotal evidence is growing that restricting calories, and fasting, activates cell-protecting mechanisms.** Research is also underway to find out whether alternate-day fasting can help reduce the risk of breast cancer.

In studies on mice with cancer, fasting appears to improve survival rates after chemotherapy. Hearing of the effects of these animal studies by Valter Longo, ten cancer patients took it upon themselves to try fasting before chemotherapy. The results were published in the medical journal *Aging*. Of these ten, the majority experienced fewer side-effects as a result of fasting than those eating normally, and the authors concluded that fasting for two to five days before chemotherapy treatment appeared to be safe. This work has yet to be taken to a truly meaningful empirical testing on humans, but it's understandable that **cancer patients are excited by the potential of calorie restriction and fasting, not least by it helping the body to mitigate the effects of cancer treatment and specifically chemotherapy.**

DETOXING

Personally, I no longer like the word "detox". It's been used and abused by marketeers in their quest to sell, sell, sell fancy products, when, in fact, detoxing is something that the body does naturally every hour of the day. However, until someone comes up with a better word, "detox" will have to do.

HOW WE BECOME TOXIC

A toxin is anything that has a detrimental effect on cell function or structure. **Toxins are materials that our bodies cannot process efficiently.** Over time they build up and, as a result, our systems function below par, leaving us drained, tired and frequently ill. People become "toxic" in many ways – through diet, lifestyle and the environment, as a natural by-product of metabolism, and through genetic lineage. Stress and harmful emotions can also create a kind of toxic environment.

Toxins include, but are not limited to:

- Food additives, flavourings and colourings.

- Household and personal cleaning chemicals, which are both inhaled and absorbed via the skin.

- Agricultural chemicals, such as pesticides, fungicides and herbicides.

- Heavy metals, which occur naturally but are poisonous.

- Oestrogens, which enter the environment due to human usage of the contraceptive pill and HRT.

- Xeno-oestrogens, which are chemicals that mimic oestrogen.

....And here are the most common ways people become toxic on the inside:

- **Eating a poor diet.** This includes low-fibre foods, fried foods and foods tainted with synthetic chemicals. Unlike live foods (fresh fruits and vegetables), these lack the enzymes that assist proper digestion and assimilation, and the fibre or bulk that assists proper elimination. They're also void of essential vitamins, minerals and other basic nutrients.

- **Eating too much.** Over-eating puts a great amount of stress on our digestive system. The body must produce hydrochloric acid, pancreatic enzymes, bile and other digestive factors to process a meal. When we over-eat, the digestive system finds it hard to meet the demands placed upon it. The stomach bloats as the digestive system goes into turmoil. Foods aren't broken down properly and tend to lodge in the lower intestine. Vital nutrients are then not absorbed.

- **Inadequate water intake.** When the body isn't receiving enough water, toxins tend to stagnate, hindering all digestive and eliminative processes.

- **Exposure to synthetic chemicals in food and environmental pollutants.** A clean, strong system can metabolize and excrete many pollutants, but when the body is weak or constipated, they're stored as unusable substances. As more and different chemicals enter the body, they tend to interact with those already there, forming second-generation chemicals that can be far more harmful than the originals.

- **Being stressed.** Stress hinders proper digestion, absorption and elimination of foods.

- **Overuse of antibiotics.** Antibiotics have a damaging effect on the intestines, especially if they're taken for extensive periods of time. Reducing the use of unnecessary antibiotics will also help minimize the very real danger of bacterial resistance.

- **Lack of exercise.** This lowers metabolic efficiency, and without circulatory stimulation, the body's natural cleansing systems are weakened.

- **Eating late at night.** The human body uses sleep to repair, rebuild and restore itself. In essence, the body uses the sleeping hours to cleanse and build. When a person goes to sleep with a full stomach, the body isn't at rest but is busy digesting and processing food. In addition, the body requires gravity to assist the passage of food from the stomach down the digestive tract.

Q *If the body detoxes itself anyway, why bother to do anything further?*

A Just as your home or office can become dusty and dirty, so your body can become clogged up with toxins and waste matter from the environment. A healthy body is able to disarm toxins by breaking them down, storing them in fat tissue or excreting them. However, here's the crux – many, if not most, people are depleted in the nutrients needed to detox optimally, and chronic health problems, sluggishness and weight gain are common results.

If you've never given your digestion much thought, don't beat yourself up about being neglectful. Unlike the head or the tips of the fingers, the gut contains very few nerve endings. What this means is, we're not so aware when things aren't working well. When you have a headache you feel every throbbing pulse and do something about it. In contrast, gut problems go unresolved and uncared for over long periods.

The good news is, when you improve digestion, a whole range of seemingly unrelated health issues can improve. For example, it's not only the job of the white blood cells (the leukocytes) to defend your body since the digestive system forms the basis of your immune system with the action of beneficial bacteria.

Improving the ecology of the gut can be achieved with a juice fast and healthy diet.

USING A JUICE FAST TO DETOX

A juice fast stands head and shoulders above other fasting techniques in its self-healing effect and is often mentioned in the context of detoxing the body.

Juice fasting is based on consuming juices and broths only, whereas intermittent fasting adds lean protein and fat for the feeling of fullness. Studies have shown that eating as little as 10g (¼oz) of essential amino acids (found in high-quality proteins) can switch off autophagy. Therefore, a juice fast is best placed to give your body a good "spring clean" because juices are typically very low in protein.

The simple act of juicing a fruit or vegetable will help you absorb more of the nutrients from it. The caveat here is that you should make the juice fresh rather than drink pasteurized fruit juice from a carton or bottle. The process of juicing eliminates a lot of the fibre that needs to be digested. Cutting out the bulk and drinking only the juice means that you can very effectively hit your *antioxidant* targets in one small cup. Juice provides tiny "particles" of nutrients that are readily absorbed into the bloodstream.

Fresh juices provide a highly effective fast-track and – importantly – easy delivery mechanism for the body to absorb and process key vitamins, minerals and plant chemicals (phytonutrients) that are so beneficial to our health. A fresh juice contains a concentration of nutrients that have been separated from pulp, making it easier to consume what's required to assist the healing process. **In essence, a fresh juice should be considered more of a body tonic than a tasty drink.**

Q *Will I get withdrawal symptons on a juice fast?*

A The folklore of fasting is littered with stories about the dramatic side-effects of a juice fast. This is usually because the contrast between the diet and lifestyle before and after is simply too great. Or, in some cases, the enterprising individual has decided to "retox", that is go on an almighty bender before entering detox – not a good idea.

One of the most dramatic side-effects I ever witnessed was when a client was coming off a 20-year-long diet cola habit during a juice-fasting retreat. Her symptoms were akin to what you'd expect from coming off a class-A drug. The rest of the detox group watched mesmerized at her descent from bubbly, bouncy guest on arrival to a sweating, vomiting, pale-faced shadow of her former self after just 24 hours of juicing. Even I was a little worried. Luckily, her troubled time was followed by a rapid and dramatic improvement two days later, at which point she declared that she felt "reborn" and would never touch a drop of cola again.

So, learn from my diet cola story and **start with a transition diet. Fasting can be a challenge physically and psychologically. I recommend having at least three days on the Countdown Plan (see page 178) to prepare. Juice fasting should be undertaken for between one and five days for optimum results – usually once or twice a year.** Any longer requires more management and should only be considered when there are adequate reserves (body fat) or if there's a specific medical condition. **Some people find that weekend-long juice fasts four times a year are helpful.**

Q *What are the most common side-effects of a juice fast?*

A **Let me be frank – a juice fast isn't a good idea for a romantic break or naughty weekend away.** During a juice fast the capacity of the eliminative organs – lungs, liver, kidneys, and skin – is greatly increased, and masses of accumulated metabolic wastes and toxins are quickly expelled. It's like pressing the accelerator button on your body's waste disposal unit. As part of the eliminative process, your body will be cleansing itself of old, accumulated wastes and toxins. This typically throws up symptoms such as offensive breath, dark urine, increased faecal waste, skin eruptions, perspiration and increased mucus. As I said, it's not exactly romantic!

Your digestive system is the star of a fasting programme. **Poor digestion can be a hidden cause of weight gain, or more accurately, water retention.** For example, if your body's responding to an allergy or intolerance it will often retain water. So, when fasting, there's often a "quick-win" water loss that equates to an extra kilo being lost.

Q *What about fibre?*

A The process of juicing extracts the pulp (fibre) of the fruits and vegetables so on a juice fast it's a good idea to restore some bulk to maintain a healthy transit of waste matter through the gastrointestinal tract. Psyllium husks, a soluble form of fibre, do just the trick as, when taken with adequate amounts of fluids, they absorb water to form a large mass. In people with constipation, this mass stimulates the bowel to move, whereas in people with diarrhoea it can slow things down and reduce bowel movements.

Some recent research also shows that psyllium husks may lower cholesterol. It's thought that the fibre stimulates the conversion of cholesterol into bile acid and increases bile acid excretion. In addition, psyllium husks may even decrease the intestinal absorption of cholesterol.

Psyllium comes from the plant *Plantago ovata* and is native to India. It is readily available in health food shops and online stores, either as husks or in powdered form. In non-fasting, normal dietary conditions, whole grains provide dietary fibre and similar beneficial effects to psyllium, so a supplement isn't needed unless recommended by your health care practitioner.

Q *Can colon cleansing help?*

A Your bowels are not just "poo pipes". Toxins and metabolic wastes from the blood and tissues are discharged into the intestinal canal to be excreted from the body. Not surprisingly, one of the long-established techniques to support the body's elimination organs during a fast is colon hydrotherapy or enemas. This is a technique that involves taking in water into the large intestine, also known as the bowel, to assist the removal of waste.

Colon hydrotherapy is not a new procedure. Enemas and rituals involving the washing of the colon with water have been used since pagan times. The first recorded mention of colon cleansing is on an Egyptian medical papyrus dated as early as 1500BCE. Ancient and modern tribes in the Amazon, Central Africa and remote parts of Asia have used river water for bowel cleansing, usually as part of magic-medical rites of passage performed by priests or shamans. Colon-cleansing therapies were an important part of Taoist training regimens and these therapies still form one of the fundamental practices of yoga teaching. Hippocrates, Galen and Paracelsus, who are recognized as the founding fathers of Western medicine, described, practised and prescribed the use of enemas for colon cleansing. In Europe and the USA, colon-cleansing treatments were popular in the early decades of the 20th century and were often performed on patients by doctors practising in sanatoria (health spas) and hospitals. From the 1920s to the 1960s, most medical practitioners were in favour of regular enemas, and these were often used as part of hospital treatment.

Having moved to the fringes of mainstream medical practice, colon hydrotherapy is now a popular holistic treatment. **As with all treatments, colon hydrotherapy should be undertaken only by a professionally trained and insured colon hydrotherapist who uses disposable equipment.** If you want to try it alongside a fasting programme, do your own research and find who you're comfortable with. In most spa-based fasting programmes, colon hydrotherapy or a self-administered method of colon cleansing such as enemas will be offered as a support to the core programme.

CHAPTER 4

EAT, FAST AND PERFORM BETTER

CAN FASTING GIVE YOU A YOUNGER BRAIN?

The potential benefits of fasting go beyond weight loss and physical health. If you've ever found yourself befuddled about where you could possibly have left your keys/phone/purse/marbles, you'll know that memory loss is a very frightening thing. The threat of long-term conditions like *Alzheimer's* is arguably one of the most worrying aspects of ageing. But there is hope. **Researchers at the National Institute on Aging in Baltimore have found evidence that fasting for one or two days each week may help protect the brain against Alzheimer's, *Parkinson's* and other brain diseases.**

ISN'T BREAKFAST IMPORTANT "BRAIN FOOD"?
Children who eat breakfast tend to perform better in cognitive tests, but this doesn't seem to be the case for adults. **Studies have shown that short-term food reduction doesn't actually impair cognitive function in adults. Prolonged dieting, on the other hand, does.** This means that the perceived deterioration in brain function may, in fact, have a psychological cause – rather than being caused by a dip in blood sugar, lack of concentration may be a result of the stress of being "on a diet" (the way it tends to make you feel grumpy, miserable, and obsessive about food). Of course, it's true that the brain uses glucose for fuel, but as we've seen in previous chapters, our bodies have enough stored glucose to see us through a short fast.

In one study, published in the *American Journal of Clinical Nutrition*, **scientists observed that fasting and non-fasting groups of adults performed similarly in cognitive tests, even after two days without food.** This is thought to relate to adaptive mechanisms – as adults, when we don't have food available, it's important that we have the mental clarity to go out and find it. Our hunter-gatherer ancestors didn't have the option to pop out to the supermarket to grab a snack, and those who could think more clearly when hungry were more likely to be able to find food or outsmart predators. This was a survival advantage, and so the genetic factors that maintained cognitive function when food was scarce were passed on. As there haven't been dramatic changes in our genes since caveman times, it makes sense that the ability to think clearly when we haven't eaten for a while should still be the norm.

FASTING AND BRAIN HEALTH

Professor Mark Mattson, a renowned researcher at the National Institute on Aging, has dedicated his career to studying the effects of fasting on brain ageing. Until now, all his research has been on mice, but there's now enough evidence of the beneficial effects of fasting on the brains of mice to begin research on humans.

At the National Institute on Aging, mice have been bred to develop a susceptibility to Alzheimer's disease. If they are then put on a "fast food" diet which is high in sugar, they experience an earlier onset of learning and memory problems. But if they're made to fast every other day, they find it much easier to remember their way around a maze. Brain scans on the mice show that fasting actually encourages new brain cells (neurons) to form by placing a mild level of stress on the brain cells, which encourages them to build up a resistance to future stress, as well as building new proteins. Other researchers have found that fasting also increases the rate of autophagy in the brain, thereby getting rid of any damaged "grey matter" and making way for healthy new cells. **So, while it's too early to tell whether fasting is the miracle cure for memory loss and age-related brain diseases, the research definitely sounds promising.**

WHAT ELSE CAN I DO TO KEEP MY BRAIN YOUNG?

Sadly, the exact reasons why some people are susceptible to diseases such as Alzheimer's are unclear. It's generally accepted that diets rich in fruit, vegetables and healthy fats from fish, avocados and olives (typically like the Mediterranean diet) are associated with good brain health. What's good for the body is also good for the brain!

One of the most important things that you can do for your body and brain is to get active and regular fasting might just help you do that. Recent studies published in the *Archives of Internal Medicine* indicate that the more active we are as we get older – even if it's just gentle walking the longer our brains will stay healthy. **It sounds like the recipe for a healthy brain could be fasting combined with an active lifestyle and a real-food based diet – just what I have in mind!**

CAN FASTING MAKE YOU FASTER?

I have to declare an interest here... For a few years I've loved the release that running has given me, especially after having my second baby. In fact, I've been a competitive soul from day dot. In my early youth I was good at badminton and represented Scotland in the game. In those days, not much attention was paid to sports nutrition, and since badminton is a largely anaerobic discipline it was possible to get by without thinking too much about what you were eating. Now, of course, everything has changed. Nutritionists feature large in all serious sport – not least, I imagine, because the "quick fix" route of banned substances has come under the spotlight, and, of course, we're all more aware of nutrition's role in exercise.

My running has become something of a "fix" – a means of releasing tension, either before the stress of the school run, or after the stress of a day's work. My usual preparation used to consist of an espresso and a mostly empty stomach. While that works for a quick half-hour run, it was only when I stepped up to training for the London Marathon in 2011 that I became more scientific and observant of my nutritional requirements. I also wondered whether fasting during training or pre-event could make a person run faster.

COMMON QUESTIONS AND ANSWERS

Q *What's the truth about sports drinks?*

A If you're a keen runner or cyclist, or harbour ambitions to run a marathon, you're probably aware of the importance of getting plenty of carbs. It's impossible to open up a running magazine or take part in a race without being bombarded with adverts for the latest energy drink or gel.

It's a fact that topping up your fuel levels with sugar – whether from fruit juice, sweets or expensive sports drinks – can make you run faster if your existing energy levels are low. Countless sports nutrition studies confirm that they do benefit performance. And the British public are buying into the dream *en masse.* In 2010, we drank 600 million litres of energy drinks and sports drinks.

However, **topping up your blood sugar during exercise is only beneficial if you're taking part in high-intensity exercise that lasts for more than an hour**, such as running a half-marathon or competing in a football match. In other cases, it won't do you any favours at all.

Q *What about fasting and exercise during Ramadan?*

A Interest in the effects of fasting on fitness has increased in recent years, inspired by studies on what happens to Muslim athletes during the month of Ramadan. During Ramadan, Muslims are required to observe a period of fasting from dawn until sunset. This includes avoiding not only food, but fluids too. As the dates of Ramadan change from year to year, this means that it can take place across major events in the sporting calendar, such as the 2012 Olympics. If you believe the sports nutrition adverts, you may think that not being able to eat or drink regularly would ruin an athlete's chances of winning, but that doesn't necessarily seem to be the case.

While most medal contenders at the 2012 Olympics seem to have taken the opportunity to postpone their fast until later in the year, in 1980 Tanzanian runner Suleiman Nyambui won silver in the 5,000 metres while observing the Ramadan fast. The effects of fasting on athletes' ability to compete and train during Ramadan are mixed. Several studies summarizing the research were published in the *Journal of Sports Science* in 2012. The overall picture was that the effects of fasting on performance are minimal, so long as overall nutritional intake and other factors, such as quality of sleep, are maintained.

Nevertheless, training while fasting – especially in the case of Ramadan, where athletes are also likely to be dehydrated through avoiding water – may make you feel more tired or reduce the amount of effort that you're able to put in. But, for mere mortals rather than Olympians, intermittent fasting has the promising ability to improve overall fitness or sports performance.

Q *Should I cut carbs?*

A As mentioned at the beginning of this chapter, the roots of how fasting may benefit performance are in our evolutionary past. Our caveman ancestors simply didn't have the opportunity to fuel up with carbohydrates before they went off to forage and hunt. Cycles of feast and famine meant that the ability to perform extended periods of physical activity on an empty stomach was an advantage when it came to survival. It's thought that our genetic make-up hasn't changed much in the 10,000 or so years since. So **it makes sense, in theory, that humans are designed to exercise without taking on extra fuel.**

At all times, our bodies burn both fat and carbohydrate for energy. While our storage capacity for carbohydrate is limited to around 500 calories-worth, most of us have more than enough fat stores to keep us going for a while. Say you're 70kg (11st) and your body fat is 25 percent – that means you have over 150,000 calories of fat in storage.

Aerobic training increases the proportion of fat to carbohydrate burned, making it easier to exercise for long periods of time. Just as the body adapts to any training stimulus by getting stronger or fitter, the idea is that training when fasting – when stored carbohydrate levels are low – stimulates the body to become even more efficient at using stored fat for fuel. While it might therefore seem like a no-brainer that exercising without extra carbohydrate will help your body adapt, it has long been recommended that endurance athletes consume a carbohydrate-rich diet.

Carbohydrate is stored in muscles as *glycogen*, where it can easily be broken down into glucose to fuel movement. **Most research continues to emphasize the importance of adequate carbohydrate intake, before, during and after exercise.** This is particularly important during high-intensity events, where glucose is the main fuel – stored fat is pretty good at fuelling slow and steady movement, but it's glucose that your body turns to when you want to move fast. In events or training that last over an hour, it's generally recommended that 30–60g (1–2¼oz) of carbohydrate is consumed per hour, in the form of drinks, gels or food.

The mistake that many of us make is to rely on topping up our carbohydrate stores *too* **much.** This could also be the reason why many people don't lose weight when they start exercising. A typical bottle of sports drink can take half an hour of leisurely cycling to burn off, so if that's all you manage, and you add in a post-workout snack too, you could even find yourself gaining weight!

Q *What happens when you train while fasting?*

A Looking back to a study carried out by the US Army in 1988, **there's no need to fear running out of glucose if you haven't**

eaten for a day. In fact, it seems to be possible to exercise for just as long after a three-and-a-half day-fast as it is after an overnight fast when working at a low intensity. Researchers in the same study found that blood glucose levels were maintained too.

In another small study published in the *Journal of Physical Activity and Health*, this time on healthy people who exercised at a relatively high intensity for an hour-and-a-half, fasting for 16–18 hours didn't impede their efforts. Interestingly, drinking a sports drink didn't make them feel or perform better either.

Meanwhile, researchers at Pennington Biomedical Research Center have discovered that **consuming carbohydrates *during* exercise can actually decrease the expression of genes that are involved in fat metabolism**. So, the more carbs you take in during exercise, the worse your body gets at tapping into its fat stores!

Sticking to plain water, or a calorie-free drink, increases the proportion of fat burned during exercise because less glucose is available. When you consume a sports drink, the glucose is rapidly delivered to your blood and provides an instant source of fuel. Without this, you need to tap into your body's fat stores.

Research by the University of Glasgow, involving 22 recreationally active males, showed that, in a one-hour cycling test after an overnight fast, those who drank a calorie-free drink burned 41 percent more fat than those who consumed a standard sports drink. It's important to note that total energy expenditure was similar between the groups but, when thinking about weight loss, it's the total amount of calories you burn that's important. Those who drank the sports drink consumed around 250 *extra* calories, almost half of what they expended. If weight loss is a goal, there's no need to take in this extra fuel during an hour of exercise.

And in another study on cyclists, published in the *Journal of Strength and Conditioning Research* in 2009, **the combination of calorie restriction and exercising while fasting led to improvements in power-to-weight ratio** (the amount of power you can produce relative to your body weight) without harming performance.

Even if you're not a keen cyclist or runner and are just looking to lose weight, getting active first thing in the morning before your breakfast could be beneficial. Research published in the *British Journal of Nutrition* showed that overweight men who walked for an hour before eating breakfast burned more fat than those who ate first. It wasn't a huge amount – an average of around an extra five grams – but that could add up over time.

Q *What's meant by "train low, race high"?*

A **"Train low" means that some training is done without carbs to encourage the body to burn fat.** As the bulk of modern sports nutrition research highlights the role of carbohydrates in enhancing performance under race conditions, the **"race high" part involves taking on standard sports drinks or gels during events.**

"Train low" training is different from simply training after an overnight fast, when muscle glycogen levels are still relatively high. Studies investigating the "train low" approach deplete participants' glycogen stores by putting them through an hour or more of aerobic training. After an hour's rest, participants then complete up to an hour of high-intensity exercise, all with only water to drink.

A recent study published in *Medicine & Science in Sports &*

Exercise, involving 14 well-trained cyclists, showed that three weeks of high-intensity training in this glycogen-depleted state was as effective in improving time-trial performance as training with normal glycogen levels, even though power output during training was lower. **Low-glycogen training led to a greater increase in the rate of fat oxidation by increasing the levels of enzymes involved in the metabolism of fat. At the same time, it led to greater resting levels of muscle glycogen after training.** What this means is that, although training with low levels of glycogen (carbohydrate) in the muscles reduced the intensity the cyclists were able to work at during training, their race performance still improved. This is likely to be because the cyclists' muscles responded to training with low fuel levels by storing more carbohydrate at rest and becoming more efficient at burning their fat stores for fuel.

Another study published in the *European Journal of Applied Physiology* found that **a factor involved in muscle synthesis was reactivated more quickly after slow and steady endurance training in the fasted state compared to in the fed state in men.**

Interestingly, most studies on low-glycogen training have been carried out on males. Energy metabolism during exercise varies between genders. A study published in *Journal of Science and Medicine and Sport* observed a greater increase in fat metabolizing enzymes for women when they trained in the fed state, suggesting that **"train low, race high" may be more appropriate for men than women.**

While there's no clear evidence that the "train low, race high" approach will benefit performance, it's worth experimenting with if you want to lose fat *and* get faster. Fitness training is about adaptation and not necessarily performing your best. By doing some high-intensity training in a fasted state you may be able to increase the level of fat-metabolizing enzymes in your muscles, meaning that you can work at a higher effort level without taking in extra carbs when racing.

All-in-all, this suggests that taking part in aerobic exercise while you're fasting should not harm your body and may even help your body adapt to training at higher intensities without relying on sports drinks for fuel. This is an especially good thing if you're a keen runner or cyclist and tend not to feel well when you take gels or energy drinks during a race.

But be careful because **training in a glycogen-depleted state has its risks.** These include increased levels of stress hormones, muscle breakdown, fatigue and lowered immune response. If, while fasting, you decide to add some endurance training to your schedule, especially at a high intensity, it's probably best, initially, to limit it to once a week. Allow plenty of time for recovery, and monitor your response, stopping if you feel unwell or fatigued.

FASTING FOR A STRONGER BODY

Weight-training enthusiasts use intermittent fasting as a technique to build lean mass and lose fat, with the goal of achieving a "shredded" or "ripped" physique. The explosion in popularity of intermittent fasting over the past few years is in part due to fitness experts such as Martin Berkhan, who designed the "Lean Gains" 16/8 hour fast. This method focuses the fast around the times you're scheduled to work out. The reason for this is that, in order to build muscle, you need to be in positive energy and protein balance *after* your workout, otherwise your muscles will be consumed for energy instead of getting bigger. Therefore, while the workout is done in the fasted state, the biggest meal of the day is right after the workout. Some people also take "branched-chain amino acid" supplements to maximize levels of growth hormone and to kick-start the muscle-building process.

The positive results posted on the Lean Gains website speak for themselves, but the technique is also backed up by scientific research. **In one study, published in the *European Journal of Applied Physiology*, male participants grew more muscle when they did their weight training in a fasted state.** This seemed to be facilitated by eating proteins and carbohydrates soon after training. Researchers concluded that fasting activated factors which stimulated muscle cell growth in response to the nutrients.

Going back to the discussion about what happens to people who exercise while fasting during the Islamic holy month of Ramadan (see pages 89–90), Tunisian researchers found that performing aerobic training in the fasted state led to greater fat loss. Although the study was very small, the **results suggest that if you're trying to shed body fat and hold on to your muscle, doing your aerobic exercise while fasting is the way to go.** During the month-long study, participants who trained before eating lost a similar amount of weight to those who trained after eating. However, those who trained after eating did not lose as much fat, and therefore their body composition didn't improve.

STRENGTH FOR WOMEN

Just because intermittent fasting was popularized by body builders doesn't necessarily mean that resistance training in the fasted state will turn women into beefcakes. To gain significant amounts of muscle, you need to train hard – lifting progressively heavier weights several days a week – and eat more calories than you burn off. **A strong, lean, toned look can still be very feminine, so do at least consider regular training with weights.**

While fasting might help you become stronger, there is some evidence that it could also make you feel a bit wobbly! In a study by Canadian researchers, healthy young women who were asked to take part in balance trials were steadier on their feet after a meal than after a 12-hour fast. This may have implications for anyone who is worried about falling – if you're exercising to build up muscle strength after an injury, for example.

FASTING AND MOTIVATION

The final motivator, when thinking about incorporating fasting with exercise, is that it could give you *more energy* to train. There are lots of arguments over whether diet or exercise is more important when it comes to losing weight.

You may be familiar with the saying "you can't out-train a bad diet". While it's probably true that exercise alone isn't going to get you the body you want if you pay no attention to what you eat, dieting without exercise isn't a good idea either. After all, exercise comes with an impressive array of health benefits itself – from heart and lung health, to stress relief, to maintaining strong bones.

When it comes to muscle strength and the way you look, exercise is the clear winner over diet. Researchers at Ann Arbor University in Michigan looked at how women's bodies responded to diet alone versus exercise alone. They found that, as expected, diet was more effective at reducing body weight, but exercise was more effective when it came to losing fat and maintaining muscle.

The thing is, getting the motivation to exercise can be hard when you're "on a diet" because you're always eating less than you're burning off and you often feel like you just don't have the energy. **The good thing about fasting is that the gaps between meals are longer so when you do eat, you get to eat more. This means that you can time your exercise around the times when you've eaten and are feeling energetic.** You're more likely to work harder!

PERFORMANCE CASE STUDIES

REAL-LIFE EXAMPLE
NAME: **Alex**

Personal trainer Alex had always done a lot of weight training and eaten well, but in November 2011 he wanted find a method of eating that would help him strip away stubborn body fat.

> *"I first heard about fasting a number of years ago and wanted to do some more research and see how it could be implemented for body composition change. I had a look online to see how others had used it for the same goals. I run a tight food schedule anyway, but wasn't getting the results I wanted. After immersing myself in the research on fasting, I decided to experiment with it. Everything I'd read indicated that it was a good way to trick the body into holding on to muscle at the same time as losing fat."*

For two months, Alex combined a strict high-protein, low-carbohydrate diet with fasting for between 16 and 20 hours a day.

The aim of this was to reduce his body fat as quickly as possible.

> *"During this fat-loss phase, I lost 3kg [7lb] in weight – all of which was fat. I maintained my muscle mass, even though I was doing less cardio exercise than usual."*

Following on from this, Alex increased both his training and carbohydrate intake – first, to train for a rowing competition and then, for a strongman competition. His aims during these phases were to maintain a reduced body fat level, and still be prepared for competition.

Alex combined three weight-training sessions a week with two cardiovascular sessions. He took a conservative approach to increasing his cardiovascular exercise by using a heart rate monitor and slowly increasing his training sessions to 45–60 minutes. Generally he trained at midday, before his main meal, and on certain days he trained early in the morning, which left him feeling quite drained by mid afternoon.

> *"I stuck to my plan rigidly most of the time. The only exceptions were at the weekend, when I sometimes had a few drinks. On Sundays, I usually had a 'cheat' meal too – a roast dinner and dessert! If anything, I think I possibly cut my calories too much in the early stages. When I started training for the rowing competition, my hunger levels spiked dramatically by the evening."*

To counteract these feelings of hunger and tiredness, Alex added some carbs after cardiovascular training – for example, a number of large bowls of porridge. To meet his calorie requirement, Alex found he was sometimes eating non-stop for an hour at a time!

Although Alex's main aim was to increase strength and improve the way he looked, he performed better than he expected in the rowing competition. He also gained strength, finding that the amount of weight he could lift went up consistently week after week, which allowed him to place well in the strongman competition, too.

> "The main benefit was that it brought me back in line with how much food I really need. The biggest strength of intermittent fasting is that it simply reduces your exposure to food. I like eating a lot when I do eat! I find that pairing intermittent fasting with low-carb food works best for me, although I suffer when I train in the early morning, and I experience an increased hunger for carbs after intense exercise. I still follow the 16–20-hour fast pattern most days but allow myself a relaxed day off on a Saturday, when I eat whatever I want to, but still keep it pretty clean."

Alex's main advice for anyone considering pairing intermittent fasting with intensive training would be:

- Stretch out the timescale – don't try to lose fat too quickly.

- If you are cutting down on carbs, do this gradually to allow your metabolism time to adapt.

- Have your main meal immediately after training.

- Have a relaxed day off once a week.

REAL-LIFE EXAMPLE

NAME: Dana

Like Alex, Dana was used to training hard, and wanted to use fasting as a method of becoming very lean. She had been working out regularly for over two years and was already fit and toned but hoped that fasting would help her get rid of the last of her belly fat!

Dana followed a strict 20-hour fast, concentrating all of her meals in a small window between 1pm and 5pm.

> *"I usually stick to it very strictly, but sometimes I extend the eating time by an hour or two if I don't get the chance to eat enough that day. Most of the time I find it hard to eat all my daily calories in only four hours. I usually break it into two main meals and a small snack if time allows. Another inconvenience is that I feel stuffed during the eating window and cannot train. I have to train only in the morning on an empty stomach, because I feel lighter and can move better."*

Dana followed this pattern for three weeks, and during this time lost 2kg (4lb).

> *"I feel lighter, my stomach is flatter and I can see results in building lean muscle."*

PART 2

MAKING FASTING WORK FOR YOU

- FIT YOU AND YOUR LIFE TO FASTING
- ME TARZAN, YOU JANE
- THE FASTING STATE OF MIND

CHAPTER 5

FIT YOU AND YOUR LIFE TO FASTING

FOOD PERSONALITIES

Let's start by talking about your food personality. Yes, you have one! Pop psychology will come up with an alarming array of traits that are determined by how you interact with your knife and fork. Here are a couple of examples:

Slow eater? "You will prioritize your own needs first."

Enjoy trying new foods? "Open-minded and will embrace change."

Let's put aside a sweeping character profile for now and focus on the big picture. We're all unique in how we relate to food, and it makes perfect sense that a fasting approach that suits one person won't suit another. For example, in my close circle of family and friends I find every conceivable food personality type:

- **Man-child** – the type of bloke who never grows up and is deeply suspicious of anything new. Still insists on cartoon character cereal and thinks nobody can match his Mum's Sunday roast (like, *never*).

- **The grab-and-go type** – thinks life's too short for proper meals and prefers, quite literally, to eat on the run, usually propped up by caffeine or sugary snacks at regular intervals.

- **The Monday dieter** – we've all been there – a few drinks after work at the end of a tough week and it's goodbye to good intentions.

- **The free spirit** – can consume anything and everything without putting on weight. Funnily enough, these types are usually slim as they don't tend to eat when they're bored or upset but simply when they're hungry.

- **Food hypochondriac** – trawls the Internet for symptom checkers in her lunch hour and is convinced she has an intolerance to most major food groups, despite being told by her doctor and nutritionist that everything is just fine.

- **Husband** – burns off all he consumes, even pastries, pies and beer at the rugby. Maddeningly healthy. It's not fair!

OK, I'm poking a little bit of fun but I bet my predicament about how to keep everyone's belly happy is similar to yours or will reflect some aspect of your upbringing.

Rather than adopt the usual "one size fits all" approach, try overlaying your personality traits with your current life circumstances to give you a more personal take on choosing which *Eat, Fast, Slim* method will suit you best.

Take a moment to write down everything you ate yesterday. How many times did you eat because your body was giving you signals that you were hungry (a rumbling tummy, for example)? What else prompted you to eat?

For example:

- "I always eat at that time."

- "I didn't want it to go to waste."

- "I couldn't resist."

Let's assume that you're motivated to give fasting a try. The next step is to find a fasting approach that will work best for you and your life. Think about it like speed dating. If the approach you choose is a bit dull, slow and doesn't quite hit the spot, say, "Thanks for the time, but no thanks" and move on!

First, let's summarize some of the main things to bear in mind:

- Men and women respond a little differently.

- Different personalities respond differently.

- Juice fasting will be best if your goal is to help heal a health condition.

- Lifestyle intermittent fasting will suit if your goal is a buff and toned body.

- If your goal is to have an overall "time-out", a retreat-based juice fast will probably suit you best.

To keep matters as simple as possible, I classify all fasting methods as either lifestyle fasts or juice fasts. Remember that whichever fasting method ends up suiting you best, it's important to follow the advice in the "Nutritional Rules for Fasting" chapter. When you eat, you must eat well. This means no cutting out of major food groups and no heavily processed foods. If you can't pronounce what it says on the label, the chances are you shouldn't be eating it.

LIFESTYLE FASTS

Lifestyle fasts are designed to be incorporated into a long-term eating pattern and have been popularized by bodybuilders and "ultra" athletes who've been switched on to fasting for years because it's incredibly good at fighting fat. Lifestyle fasts are also popular among celebrities or the uber health-conscious in search of the body beautiful.

Intermittent fasting is a popular type of lifestyle fasting and usually means leaving a long gap between one meal and the next at least once a week. With some plans you skip a couple of meals randomly once or twice a week, or there again you might eat only during a four- to eight-hour window every day, fasting the rest of the time.

There are many variations on this intermittent fasting theme. At the time of writing, many people are talking about the **5/2 fast**, where you dramatically restrict your calories just two days a week. During those two days you'll eat around 500 calories. Another method uses the same framework but increases the fasting day frequency to every other day.

And for years fitness buffs have used another method, known as **16/8 intermittent fasting**, to help them achieve a lean and toned body. It's really straightforward... All you have to do is skip a meal – breakfast or dinner – and ensure that what you eat most of the time is healthy.

In most cases, it will take a while to find a pattern that suits

you best. The plan on page 179 shows you an example of how to structure a week of intermittent fasting using the 16/8 method and on page 180 you'll find a plan for the 5/2 method. In both cases you can follow it exactly or adopt a variation that suits your lifestyle – after all, the point is to integrate fasting into your life, not to let fasting rule your life!

Fasting every other day (often referred to as alternate-day fasting), is a pretty tough call – 500–600 calories does not amount to much food, and it can be difficult to reach your nutritional needs on this. In fact, I'd only suggest this method if someone had to lose a lot of weight very quickly for medical reasons. From a nutritional point of view, it would require some supplement support.

For fasting purists, there is also **water fasting**, usually for a full 24 hours once a week. On this kind of fast you eat nothing but remain hydrated by sipping water throughout the day. However, this isn't easy and, in my personal opinion, not to be recommended. For this reason it's not one of my fasting protocols.

It's not all about hard work though. There's a trend among lifestyle-fasting devotees to have a "cheat day" once a week. By all means, if you'd like to relax a bit at the weekend or have the occasional day off, this will do you no harm and may even make fasting easier to stick to. But be warned – it's easy to undo all your hard work if you allow yourself to overdo it or eat all the wrong things. Stick to the nutrition rules as closely as you can *most* of the time.

If you're exercising, the generally accepted recommendation for men is that the main meal of the day is immediately after your workout, as this seems to be best for gaining muscle mass and burning fat. For women there's some evidence to suggest that training after a meal is more beneficial.

ARE YOU A LIFESTYLE FASTER?

To discover whether lifestyle fasting will suit you, tick all the statements below that you agree with:

- My main aim is to get rid of my muffin top/bingo wings/moobs/ beer belly.

- I'd like to build muscle or look more "toned".

- I've tried lots of weight-loss plans but always fall off the wagon.

- I'm looking for a straightforward eating plan that I can stick to long term.

- I feel comfortable with the idea of skipping meals.

If you counted three or more ticks, there's a good chance that lifestyle fasting will suit you. If not, move on to the section on Juice fasts (see page 112).

If you think lifestyle fasting is for you, use the next set of questions to help you decide on the frequency and length of the gaps between your meals:

1 **When do you tend to feel most hungry?**
   a) In the morning.
   b) In the afternoon or evening.
   c) My appetite varies from day to day.

2 **How big are your meals?**
   a) I tend to eat a substantial lunch and dinner.

b) I like a big breakfast, then tend to eat smaller meals later on.

c) I'm more of a grazer, and rarely eat large meals.

3 **What's a typical lunchtime like for you?**
   a) I often have an early lunch because I've skipped breakfast.
   b) I have time to make lunch my main meal of the day.
   c) I rarely have time for a proper lunch.

4 **What's a typical evening like for you?**
   a) I eat dinner with my family or partner.
   b) I grab something "on the run" and rarely eat at the table.
   c) There's no such thing as typical, but I tend to eat out at least once a week.

If you answered mostly:

a) **Try the 16/8 Lifestyle Fast, skipping breakfast daily.** With this plan you eat during an eight-hour "window" every day. Most people find that having an early lunch around 12pm works well. This means that you can have your dinner between 7pm and 8pm.

b) **Try the 16/8 Lifestyle Fast, skipping dinner.** The sample plan (see page 179) is based on lunch, dinner and a substantial afternoon snack. However, choosing to skip your evening meal instead of breakfast is also fine and may suit your lifestyle better. If this is the case, in order to make sure that you are eating enough overall and that your meals are balanced, I suggest that you use a dinner recipe at lunchtime, and have an extra snack in the afternoon just before you begin your fast. Time your eight-hour eating "window" from whenever you have breakfast. So if, for example, you have breakfast at 8am, your last meal of the day should be before 4pm. It's up to you whether you choose to have an early lunch and a substantial afternoon snack, or have a substantial snack mid-morning and save your lunch until 3pm. You may need to experiment to work out what works best for you. And remember, it's never a good idea to drink alcohol on an empty stomach, so choose another pattern if you ever drink alcohol in the evening.

c) **Try the 5/2 Lifestyle Fast.** With this pattern, you eat "normally" five days a week – in the sample plan (see page 180) there are three meals and two snacks, but feel free to pick the number of meals that suits you best. On the other two days, you're restricted to two very small meals, adding up to a total of 500–600 calories. This works well if your lifestyle is more erratic – you just need to make sure that your "fast" days are separated by at least one day.

You can effectively carry on with any of these fasting patterns for as long as you like. You can follow them for several weeks or months to help you reach a goal weight, or continue with them long term, based on whatever feels right for you and your body. **But stop if you have health issues, are underweight, are actively trying to conceive or are pregnant.** Women may want to take a break from lifestyle fasting schedule the week before their period begins as it can be harder to stick to at this time.

You'll find sample fasting plans and a wide selection of recipes in the final part of the book (see pages 176–285).

JUICE FASTS

Juice fasting comes from the tradition of the healing arts, such as naturopathy, nutritional medicine and cleansing. Fat loss is considered more of a welcome side-effect to the dynamic and often dramatic improvements to troublesome health conditions. A typical juice fast day consists of five juices and a broth, spread evenly throughout the day.

Aside from what passes your lips, the main practical difference between a juice fast and intermittent fasting is the length of time you do them for – juice fasts are short term only. However, there are other differences too. **The perfect conditions in which to undertake a juice fast involve plenty of rest and relaxation in order to create the right internal environment for self-healing.** During a juice detox your body is working hard to heal and rejuvenate and so the maxim "less is more" applies here – if you can, ditch the spinning class in favour of a spa treatment.

Ideally, follow a juice fast for between one and five days. The first two days are generally the hardest but it's worth persevering for at least three days to get the best result. After many years of working with juice fasting, I've come to the conclusion that the optimum period on this type of fast is generally just short of five days. Any longer requires more management and should only be considered when there are adequate reserves (body fat) or if there's a specific medical condition – although losing the typical 2.25kg (5lb) safely in less than a week by doing a juice fast can feel fantastic!

For many people, weekend-long juice fasts every three months are a popular addition to an annual five-day juice-fast. This means that the next boost is never more than a season away and you have a regular time to focus on you and your body. A typical juice-fast day consists of five juices and a broth, spread evenly throughout the day.

There are some contra-indications to juice fasting for certain medical conditions so make sure you read the "Fasting Safely" chapter before getting started.

ARE YOU A JUICE FASTER?

To see if juice fasting is for you, tick all the statements below that you agree with:

- My main aim is to improve the symptoms of a health condition.

- I'm concerned about the effects of ageing on my health.

- I'd find it very difficult to skip meals regularly.

- I can set aside between one and five days to dedicate to juicing and relaxation.

- I'm looking for a "kick start" to weight loss and I'd like to see a quick result.

If you count three or more ticks, there's a good chance that a short-term juice fast will suit you. You'll find a Juice Fast plan on page 182) and a wide selection of recipes on pages 276–85).

SUPPORTING A JUICE FAST

Many juice-fasting programmes take place in a spa environment with saunas, relaxing massage and activities such as yoga built into the day. Granted, this can be hard to emulate at home. I've attempted many an ill-thought-through juice fast at home, only to be thwarted by a toddler knocking over my hard-earned (and time-consuming) juice, or worse, finding that my day's quota of juices has been raided by a thirsty teenage son and his mates after school. (In the end, he was assigned his own fridge!)

So, if you can create a bubble in which to **enjoy some "me time" during a juice fast**, all the better. Book up a massage, visit the sauna or steam room at the local gym and generally prioritize your well-being in the broadest sense. (If all else fails, join me on one of my juice fasting retreats!)

It's important to think ahead before you begin your first juice fast in order to get the most out of the experience by minimizing negative side-effects. This means getting your nutrition basics right *before* you begin. The simplest way to do this is to first follow my Countdown Plan (see page 178) for at least three days, to make sure that you're abiding by the rules in the "Nutritional Rules for Fasting" chapter.

There's one area of supporting a juice fast that requires a different kind of intervention. During a juice fast you don't take in bulk (bulk usually helps to move the indigestible food residue and the body's own wastes toward the exit), but you may wish to support the process of bowel elimination in a different way by colon cleansing (see pages 83–4).

FASTING AND THE "REAL WORLD"

What I love about fasting compared to pretty much any other diet is its simplicity. It's much easier to stick to something that is more about watching the clock than counting every calorie. It's a healthy, simple answer in an industry that has become tricky, over-complicated and sometimes just downright ridiculous (more on that in a minute). The fact of the matter is if a weight-loss claim sounds too good to be true, it probably is. No fad diet is practical in terms of everyday life and is therefore highly unlikely to be sustainable in the long term. That's why the nutritional rules and fasting plans that you'll find in *this* book are firmly rooted in sound healthy eating principles.

THE FASTER'S FRIENDS AND FOES

Fasting is inherently easy to follow but – no matter which fasting plan you choose – you still need to guard against things in life that can trip you up, distract you from your goal and spiral you into self-sabotage. I call them the "faster's foes" and, needless to say, those old vices of greed and temptation figure large.

The people you spend your time with, how well you sleep and the food you choose to eat play a huge part in how easily you fit fasting into your life. The so-called "faster's friends" are the people, habits and things that you can always draw on for support, so make sure you read "The Fasting State of Mind" chapter so that you are mentally prepared.

Most important of all is what you choose to eat outside your fasting hours. The advice in the "Nutritional Rules for Fasting" chapter is essential reading, and the Fasting Plans (see pages 178–82) will help make sensible eating easier for you.

Last but not least, **there's the silly stuff you really *don't* need...**

GIMMICKS ON TRIAL

While you're trying to find your way in fasting, you may come across a lot of weird and wonderful advice. In fact, we have a board on the wall in the office where my rather acerbic team gather some of the stranger admonitions and homilies from around the world of diet fads and brands. If you're reading this book in order to lose weight, I'm pretty sure it won't be the first book you've ever read on the subject (and perhaps you've already encountered some of the strange diets out there that could put your health – and your sanity – at risk). **Below are some fun snippets that illustrate just what nonsense is out there.**

> *"If you can find rabbit, it is an excellent source of pure protein. But do not add mustard sauce on Thursdays."*
> **The Dukan Diet** by Dr Pierre Dukan (Hodder & Stoughton, 2010, p.143)

> *"You eat nine specially-formulated cookies (just 60 calories each) throughout the day to keep hunger away."*
> **The Cookie Diet** (www.cookiediet.com)

> *"Eat absolutely no fruit, bread, pasta, grains, starchy vegetables or dairy products other than cheese, cream or butter. [...] Eat nothing that is not on the acceptable foods list."* [The acceptable foods list includes such delights as pheasant, veal and flounder!]
> **Dr Atkins New Diet Revolution** by Robert C. Atkins, MD (Ebury Press, 1992, p.123)

> *"The combination of no breakfast, a cold bath and a caffeine boost is powerful. [...] If you hate black coffee, use caffeine pills."*
> **Six Weeks to OMG** by Venice A. Fulton (Michael Joseph, 2012, pp.64–5)

COLD BATHS AND CAFFEINE

Cold baths are harmless but a bit daft in daily life. I've used cold baths in the past for post-marathon training soaks (so-called "nature's anti-inflammatory") and in that context they may have a place. However, depending on them to boost your weight loss isn't a sensible strategy. Any extra calories burned when your body raises its core temperature will most likely be used up by the splash of milk you put in your hot tea or coffee to warm up again. In other words, in terms of calorie burn, sitting in a cold bath has a negligible effect. If you want to invigorate yourself in the morning in a more pleasant way, simply have a blast of cold after a warm shower. It's certainly good for circulation and some people even claim that it gives hair an extra shine.

Now, I love a cup of java as much as the next person but using excessive amounts of caffeine to increase calorie burn alongside fasting isn't likely to help either. As anyone who has lived through a student "all-nighter" essay deadline knows, caffeine is great at boosting mental alertness and abating drowsiness due to its effect on the central nervous system. However, pull this trick too often and caffeine becomes the enemy of a sound night's sleep. Inadequate sleep, which all of us experience from time to time, makes good intentions so easily slip away in favour of a quick-fix carb.

Therefore, the rule is that a little caffeine is fine but a lot isn't. It's also addictive (come off it for a day and feel those headaches), so keep your coffee quota to no more than two small cups a day – no super-sized lattes! You could even try switching to the infinitely more healthy green tea –although it contains some caffeine it also has high levels of polyphenols, which have anti-cancer properties.

CHAPTER 6

ME TARZAN, YOU JANE

HOW MEN AND WOMEN RESPOND DIFFERENTLY TO FASTING

Our cavemen ancestors lived a very different life to us. There's debate among anthropological researchers, but it's generally believed that men were responsible for going out to hunt down dinner, while women stayed at home to look after the cave and the family. When food was in short supply, the hunters would have had to go the extra mile to catch a buffalo (or any other edible creature). They needed to be strong when food was scarce. People who could run fast and fight hard on an empty stomach were more likely to survive and pass on these abilities to future generations.

Some researchers have raised concerns about the effects of fasting on women's health, in particular their fertility. Intuitively, this view makes sense, because if very little food was available, creating another mouth to feed would have made things even more difficult for those cavemen ancestors of ours. That's how the theories go, but it's important that we put them into the context of current research before making specific recommendations.

RESEARCH FINDINGS
Here's what research has to say:

- In one study by scientists at the National Institute on Aging in the USA, male rats that were fasted intermittently for six months behaved in similar ways to those that weren't fasted. Their movement patterns and brain performance stayed the same.

- Female rats that were fasted were more alert during their normal sleep times, performed better in mental tests, and tended to move around more. Their adrenal glands (which make stress hormones) also grew.

- Forty-two percent of the female rats that were fasted developed menstrual irregularities, and in 2 percent the menstrual cycle ceased. However, female rats on a low-calorie diet (40 percent fewer calories than they needed, which is equivalent to a 1,200-calories-a-day diet for a typical woman), fared worse – 91 percent of them stopped having a menstrual cycle. This simply suggests that calorie restriction can have a negative effect on fertility.

- Studies on women indicate that fasting could lead to small differences in the levels of hormones that trigger egg maturation and release, although most women maintain a normal menstrual cycle even when fasting for two to three days at a time.

- As already discussed in the "Eat, Fast and Perform Better" chapter, there's some evidence that women's muscles respond better to training after eating than when they have fasted, whereas studies suggest that men can perform just as well if they train *before* eating.

- One study on alternate-day fasting, carried out at Pennington Biomedical Research Center in the USA, observed a reduction in insulin sensitivity and a decrease in glucose tolerance in women, while the response of men's metabolisms was all positive. However, a more recent study published in the *International Journal of Obesity*, involving 107 overweight women, found that women who fasted two days a week saw greater improvements in their insulin sensitivity over six months than those who simply cut calories. So, the jury's still out on this one.

- In other human studies, there don't appear to be any major differences between how men and women react to fasting.

Put simply, it seems that fasting can help men to run fast and lift heavy things and may help women to think clearly. The downside is that fasting may not benefit fertility, and shouldn't be combined with a diet based on foods that send blood sugar soaring. But do take note that most of these studies were small – the gender differences in how our bodies respond simply haven't been well researched.

So, what does all this mean for how men and women should approach fasting?

FASTING FOR WOMEN

Male readers, we are about to get into a bit of girl chat. Keep reading if you want an insight into how the female body works – women love a man who is sensitive to their needs! On the other hand, if you're more comfortable reading about football and beer, you'll find that kind of thing on pages 130–4.

As we've seen from the research, there's some evidence that extreme dieting can affect fertility but, notably, human studies suggest that being overweight can affect fertility too. **If you're thinking of becoming pregnant, fasting isn't automatically ruled out, but it's important to monitor any changes in your menstrual cycle during fasting and to stop once you are actively trying to conceive.**

One key difference between men and women which can affect the response to fasting is the impact of women's fluctuating hormones on mood and food choices during the menstrual cycle. **Understanding the menstrual cycle and how it impacts on cravings, weight gain and mood can be hugely empowering for women.**

I'm often asked by women why, at certain times in a woman's cycle, the scales remain "stuck" – or worse, why several pounds appear overnight – in spite of efforts to eat well. The answer is that the hormonal fluctuations your body experiences throughout the month affect your appetite and fluid retention, which naturally leads to fluctuations in weight.

In the first half of your cycle, the levels of *estradiol,* a type of oestrogen, slowly rise. Studies suggest that when oestrogen levels are high, appetite tends to be lower. This is one of the reasons why the menopausal transition, when circulating oestrogen levels fall, has been linked with weight gain. It also suggests that **a few days after your period could be the best time to begin a weight-loss plan. This is also the best time to consider fasting.**

In contrast, the appetite increases after ovulation. Researchers at the University of Ottawa looked at ten different studies of energy intake across the menstrual cycle. They found that women ate 87–500 extra calories a day, on average, in the second half of their menstrual cycle! However, this didn't have a significant effect on weight because metabolic rate is thought to increase to compensate for extra intake.

An important point to note, though, is that the women studied weren't actively trying to lose weight. The effects of the menstrual cycle on the rate of weight loss haven't been studied. Intuitively, it seems likely that a greater rate of weight loss can be achieved in the first half of the month. And it's important not to be hard on yourself if the scales appear to be "stuck" in the latter two weeks.

Fluid retention is often a factor in weight gain. The reason why women accumulate fluid before their period is unclear but it's thought to be hormonal. However, eating too many processed foods (high in salt and refined carbohydrates) may make the problem worse, and yet those are exactly the types of food we crave at this time!

THE MONTHLY CYCLE

Being aware of the effects of your menstrual cycle on your weight is the first step to overcoming the difficulties it poses. Let's look at exactly what happens to a woman's body, mind and, most importantly, appetite over the course of the 28-day cycle. This information will help you work out when and how to incorporate fasting into your lifestyle in the long term.

DAY 1

Your levels of *progesterone* (the hormone that builds up your womb lining) and oestrogen have fallen to their lowest levels and your period starts today, bringing relief from PMS symptoms. Drink plenty of water to stay hydrated and relax on the sofa with a warming cup of raspberry leaf or ginger tea.

DAY 2

This first half of your cycle is called the follicular phase and your oestrogen levels are rising. If your period is heavy, eat iron-rich foods – with a source of vitamin C to aid absorption – to keep up your energy. Try a tasty lean beef salad with spinach and orange pieces, sprinkled with sunflower seeds.

DAY 3

It's normal to feel tired during your period so try to steer clear of sugar this week – otherwise, after the initial blood sugar surge, you'll feel even more fatigued than you did before.

DAY 4

You may be feeling better, less bloated and want to get more active. Do some energizing, gentle exercise, such as yoga (although don't do inversions until your period is over), t'ai chi, Pilates or qi gong, rather than intense exercise.

DAY 5

This is a good day to start preparing for your chosen fasting regime. Clear all the junk food out of your cupboards, plan your menu for the week and stock up on healthy ingredients.

DAY 6

Your endometrium (womb lining) has already started to build up again but you should now be feeling less "hormonal", so today's a good day to begin fasting. **If you're following the 5.2 Fast, try a 500-calorie day today.**

DAY 7

Chances are you'll be feeling calmer and less stressed now your period is over, meaning cravings should be easier to resist. Use this to your advantage and eat super healthily this week by loading up on fresh vegetables and fruit and saying "no" to sugary cakes and biscuits.

DAY 8

You're at your least "hormonal" so you may be feeling level headed and prepared to tackle a big project. Cook double the amount of your favourite healthy meals and freeze the leftovers for later in your cycle when your willpower is ebbing. **Today is also a good day for your second 500-calorie day if you're following the 5/2 fast.**

DAY 9

You may notice a surge in your energy levels today as your body prepares to ovulate. This is a great week to ramp up your aerobic exercise or even to start a new activity.

DAY 10

Your oestrogen levels are rising, and your body will also produce more *follicle stimulating hormone (FSH)* and *luteinizing hormone (LH)*, which encourage your ovary to release an egg. Studies on fasting in women have shown a trend toward lower levels of these hormones when you fast, which is one of the reasons you are advised to stop fasting if you are trying to become pregnant.

DAY 11

The dramatic rise in oestrogen before ovulation may make you feel sexier, flirtier and more confident today. Make the most of it by cooking a romantic meal!

DAY 12

If you have a 28-day cycle, your oestrogen levels will reach a peak today. You may notice that your appetite is lower than usual so **this is another good day to fast.**

DAY 13

You may get slight cramps in your lower abdomen, called *Mittelschmerz*, as your ovaries are preparing to release an egg. Your ovaries will release about 500 mature eggs over the course of your lifetime – a fraction of the two million you were born with.

DAY 14

You will ovulate around now (your ovaries release a mature egg 11–16 days before your period begins). After the egg is released, it starts its journey down the fallopian tube to the uterus, which takes three to four days.

DAY 15

You may feel a little warmer. This is because your body temperature rises by about 1°C (1.8° F), after ovulation due to raised progesterone levels. Your senses will also be heightened, so indulge in a deliciously sensual meal such as a lean, organic steak or a smooth mushroom risotto.

DAY 16

The second half of your cycle, after ovulation, is called the luteal phase. This is when your progesterone levels rise and oestrogen levels start to fall. Only one small study on fasting has been carried out during the luteal phase. It lowered LH and FSH levels, but it's normal for these to fall during this phase of your cycle.

DAY 17

Increased progesterone levels this week can cause your bowel to get a bit sluggish. Combat constipation with high-fibre foods, such as beans and lentils, broccoli and cabbage, berries, apples and wholegrains such as whole-wheat pasta.

DAY 18

Your breasts may be feeling tender, and may even have increased in size slightly because your body is producing more progesterone. Although one study on fasting during this phase of your cycle showed there was no effect on progesterone levels, fasting did lower another hormone called leptin, which helps you to feel full. If you're fasting and find that your appetite is starting to become insatiable, consider limiting your fasts to days 1–15, or incorporating some juices to keep your leptin levels up.

DAY 19

If you're already dreading those pre-menstrual headaches, cut out chocolate, oranges and red wine in the week before your period. Some people find that corn, wheat and eggs may worsen hormonal headaches, so try cutting down on these just before your period is due.

DAY 20

You may be noticing PMS symptoms today, such as irritability, bloating, headaches and tearfulness. Eat plenty of wholegrains this week – a study found that eating small amounts of wholegrain carbohydrates every three hours and within an hour of going to bed helped reduce PMS symptoms in 70 percent of women. Smoothies may also help.

DAY 21

If you suffer from pre-menstrual bloating, cut down on salt in your diet as salt can cause your body to hold on to more fluid. Steer clear of processed foods and ready meals, which are often high in salt, and drink plenty of water throughout the day to help your kidneys flush more fluid through your system.

DAY 22

Levels of *serotonin*, your body's feel-good chemical, may start to fall around now. Snack on a banana, which contains the amino acid tryptophan, a building block for serotonin. Other foods containing tryptophan are free-range turkey, flaxseeds, buckwheat (great for making crêpes) and oily fish.

DAY 23

Avoid making any major decisions or hitting the high street for a shopping session as hormonal changes could cloud your judgement and make you more prone to feeling upset or angry. You're also more sensitive to pain at this stage of your cycle, so don't book in any dental appointments, leg-waxing or eyebrow-shaping treatments!

DAY 24

Are you experiencing unbearable cravings for sweet and fatty carbs? Have plenty of healthy, filling snacks to hand – plant-based proteins can be particularly good at beating cravings. Eat crunchy fresh vegetables with a hummus dip or spread oatcakes with low-fat cream cheese, and satisfy a sweet tooth with a dried fruit and nut mix.

DAY 25

Your skin may be feeling greasier and seem more clogged than normal due to lower oestrogen levels which can increase the amount of sebum or oils produced by your skin. Cleanse twice daily with a product designed for sensitive skin and keep up your water intake – aim for around 2 litres (70fl oz /8 cups) a day.

DAY 26

You may start getting cramps a day or two before your period starts. Eat a couple of servings of oily fish this week – studies have shown that women who have a high intake of omega-3 essential fatty acids (EFAs) – found in salmon, sardines and mackerel, for example – tend to have milder menstrual symptoms. EFAs also act as hormone regulators.

DAY 27

Your PMS will be reaching its peak. Add plenty of green vegetables to your shopping basket since they're high in calcium, magnesium and potassium. These crucial minerals can help calm your nervous system and reduce irritability as well as help to relieve the spasms that lead to painful cramps. A green vegetable juice is also a good idea.

DAY 28

As you wait for your period to start, you may be feeling fragile, both emotionally and physically. Eat warming, comforting foods that are easy to digest, such as porridge, soups with sweet potato or barley, a baked apple or a casserole. Spoil yourself with a cosy evening in and get an early night.

TOP TIPS:

- Start fasting a few days after your period.

- Take note of where you are in your cycle when you weigh yourself. In the two weeks before your period, don't be disheartened if the scales are stuck or you gain a pound or two. Focus on how your weight is changing from month to month.

- Use body composition scales, which measure body water percentage, as these will help you to identify whether changes in your weight are due to fluid retention.

- Make sure that you have plenty of healthy snacks to hand in the second half of your cycle, in order to avoid binging on sugary, fatty snacks after a fasting period. Prepare chopped veggies in advance, stock your fridge with reduced-fat natural yogurt, and carry nuts or oatcakes in your handbag.

- If you experience sweet cravings, have a fruit smoothie. Smoothies contain a mix of simple sugars and complex carbohydrates. In one study, these were found to reduce the severity of PMS and blunt cravings for sugary, fatty foods. So if you decide to do the 5/2 fast, you could have a smoothie in place of one of your meals.

- If you're very active, time your workouts in between meals. For example, if you are following the 16/8 fast, exercise during the early evening, before dinner. If you're following the 5/2 fast, limit exercise on 500-calorie days and wait at least until your breakfast has settled on the following day before working out.

- Take a break from fasting, or switch to a different pattern, if you notice any disturbance in your menstrual cycle.

FASTING FOR MEN

According to the Urban Dictionary, "male fasting" should not be confused with "man fasting", which is:

> *"The act of purging the male species from your life in every way for a defined amount of time..."*

While this may sound fabulous post-heartbreak or when the World Cup is on, it's not exactly practical. No, what we are talking about is the fast-becoming-popular world of fasting for weight loss and body shape change by men.

A mate of mine, in the very buff and chiselled form of Alex Smith, lives and breathes an approach to life which could best be described as measured – literally. A personal trainer by profession, Alex is an intense and very potent living proof of what intermittent fasting can do.

Every day, he follows a plan which sees him measure *to the gram* his nutrients and calories for the day, and the caloric burn of his planned activity. This sounds like serious stuff, no question, but he's pretty phlegmatic:

> *"It's no different than planning what buses or trains you're going to take!"*

Intermittent fasting plays a big role in Alex's approach:

"Sure, I'm slightly retentive about this, but there's no question about the results – a planned diet with intermittent fasting applied achieves big results, especially for my male clients who like the defined, scientific, goal-based approach to getting 'weight loss done', as many of them put it."

MEN *ARE* DIFFERENT!

Ever since Eve chose to lure the characteristically easy-to-persuade Adam in the Garden of Eden, women have known that there's a whole world of difference between the male psyche and the female psyche when it comes to self-image, eating and approaches to changing said issues.

Says one good friend of mine:

"My husband thinks that his diet is fine, thank you very much. How? Fine means that he has peas with his fish and chips, and onion rings on the side. He says that the rest of his five a day comes from grapes, which just happen to have made their way into a bottle of wine."

My own brother is even worse. His vegetable quota comes from onion rings and potatoes. If you mentioned fasting, like many men he'd think of this as his annual New Year "detox", which amounts to "going on the wagon" for five days after the excesses of the festive period.

As for body image, asking around a number of younger and middle-aged men, the only thing the former want *less* of is a lardy stomach, while the only thing the latter want *more* of is hair on the top of their head.

But it's wrong to generalize. There's no questioning the fact that male vanity publishing – think *Men's Health* magazine – has had a big impact on men's self-image and aspirations. In recent years, awareness of the benefits of living healthily has increased and more older men – I call them M.A.M.I.L.s (middle-aged men in lycra) – are participating in public running, triathlon, adventure racing and cycling events. Perhaps it's just a matter of making dieting a more attractive proposition than meeting down at the community centre each week for a ritualistic weigh-in.

Certainly, if you're a man under the age of 30, it would seem that dieting is still rarely associated with "things I need to do". However, dieting for men is coming into its own as a different section of male society – those reaching middle age and gaining responsibilities such as parenthood – contemplate what I will label "the call of mortality", or, more simply, "the male menopause" (previously known as the "mid-life crisis"). For other men, it's the unwanted appearance of breasts ("man-boobs" or "moobs") and an embarrassing belly that spurs them to take action.

In the past, doing something about weight loss might have involved some half-hearted trips to the gym and cutting down on the beer, strategies that were hardly likely to succeed or deliver lasting results. The alternatives involved constant hunger, unappetizing meal replacement shakes and tiresome calorie counting. Fasting, however, provides men with a whole new approach to losing weight and shaping up. It especially appeals to men who are concerned that dieting will make them look puny since **a recent study shows that intermittent fasting can preserve muscle mass and even support body-building trends for that *Men's Health* "ripped look".**

If you haven't done so already, read more about the various fasting methods and find your optimum fasting schedule in

the "Fit You and Your Life to Fasting" chapter. Careful though, Tiger… Rome wasn't built in the proverbial day. Many men I know are all-or-nothing, black-and-white types. **Fasting can represent a big change for most people, so take it slowly!**

THE CHALLENGES OF FASTING FOR MEN

As part of my research I asked a couple of male friends to try out fasting. There were some interesting questions thrown my way:

Q *Sounds great… so by missing a few meals I can look like a men's fitness cover model?*

A Not quite, my eager friend. Fasting requires good food choices, not diving into the nearest fast-food outlet or speed dialling the pizza delivery number at the end of every fasting period. However, my menus and recipes will keep you on the straight and narrow.

Q *I'm impatient — how long before I get results?*

A Patience, as I hope your mother told you, is a virtue. The biggest challenge will invariably be breakfast, which to most men is as vital a daily habit as reading the sports pages. Don't worry, the breakfast pangs subside after two weeks, and you'll start seeing results in your weight and shape very quickly.

Q *Calorie counting is not for me*

A Many men don't like the idea of counting calories (seeing this, wrongly, as a "girly" pursuit). If you're of this persuasion, the 16/8 lifestyle fasting technique is more likely to appeal to you than the 5/2 fast because it's based on meal skipping rather than counting calories. The 16/8 pattern was popularized by male body-builders and pretty much seems to fit the male mind-set. Alternatively, you could try a short blast of juice fasting to get quick and safe results with no need to calorie count.

Q *I'm rubbish at sticking with a diet plan. How am I going to manage?*

A Even if you're only restricting or cutting calorie intake intermittently, some of you will find it a challenge, especially if you lead a road warrior lifestyle, love your treats and have a sweet tooth, or work out a lot. My advice is to find simple ways of eating properly, planning meals and then just cutting out certain mealtimes. So long as you follow the nutrition rules you'll be just fine.

CHAPTER 7

THE FASTING STATE OF MIND

FEELING "CONNECTED"

When I decided to write this book I promised myself that I wouldn't shy away from something that science, or nutrition for that matter, will never be able to pin down or explain – what fasting *feels* like, or how *connected* it can make you feel – but describing this is nigh on impossible.

So, let me start with a story instead... Once upon a time an Indian guru was asked what the difference was between wellness and illness. The wise man went up to a blackboard and wrote the word "illness". He circled the first letter, "i", and then he wrote the word "wellness" and circled the first two letters, "we".

Fasting helps you connect better with yourself. If your body is your vehicle, your mind is surely your driver. **Fasting also helps people to connect better with each other**, and anything that creates a sense of connection will surely be healing.

"KNOW THYSELF"

When trying to explain how to cultivate a fasting state of mind, the ancient Greek aphorism, "know thyself", seems like a perfect place to start, but this can be trickier than it sounds. In our busy world, with all its digital chatter, noise, pressure and expectations, if you ask a person to name something they would really like, it's quite likely to be some superficial, material object. However, more often than not, people (my husband included) express their heart's desire as a negative – for example, "less pressure/stress".

Time after time in my clinics, workshops and retreats I've seen that getting beneath the surface of polite, bland sound bites requires sensitive probing and perseverance. I've often found that this is where fasting can help. During a fast, emotions that have long been buried can come to the surface, often with more urgency and force than expected. At first, this may simply be the person rebelling against having limited food, even if the fast is self-inflicted – a bit like your toddler-self, stomping your little feet when you were told, "No, you can't have that lolly"!

Gradually though, fasting can be like a release. I liken it to leaving a door ajar in the brain for emotions to escape. It doesn't mean you fall to your knees, wailing about your first heartbreak or rejection. I've found that it's much more subtle and much more healing than that. After all, **fasting has a purpose and has been used for thousands of years to gain spiritual insight and connect with the unseen, whatever that means to you.**

Back in the day, fasting usually took place in a remote place where the person could spend time alone. The mind experience of fasting, just like the body experience, has to be created, or at least permitted. It's not always practical to do this, of course. We can't suddenly renounce our worldly goods and become a wandering mystic just because we've had a tough Tuesday at work!

At the most basic level, **one thing that fasting does for the mind is to make you much more conscious of what you *are* eating.** If you haven't eaten for 16 hours you'll savour your first mouthful – I guarantee it!

MEDITATION

For those with ambition above and beyond the physical benefits of fasting, **getting into the fasting state of mind can be helped by**

meditation, and if you have the time and inclination at least once in your life, a week's retreat can take the fasting experience to another level.

Meditation can be viewed in scientific terms for its effects on the mind and the body. During meditation, a marked increase in blood flow slows heart rate, and high blood pressure drops to within normal ranges. Recent research indicates that meditation can also boost the immune system and reduce *free radicals* – in effect, a slowing down of the ageing process.

There's much talk about the power of meditation and how you can use your mind to manifest great piles of money. But, becoming more aware of your mind is not just about manipulating it or attempting only to have positive thoughts – rather, it's about the ability to direct your attention toward or away from the mind at will.

My most intensive fast was on a 10-day silent meditation retreat during my time in India. One evening, five days into the experience when I was seriously doubting my judgement about freezing my butt off in a cold cave in the Himalayas, I had what I've come to realize was a "breakthough" moment. In spiritual terms I'd describe it as a moment of grace. With a raw, pure energy of infinite magnitude, my mind flashed through formative experiences – good and bad – that had shaped my life. As my mind was swept along on this emotional rollercoaster, my body conveniently left the room, leaving me nowhere to run or hide... or at least that was how it felt!

Even more strangely (and I realize I may lose a few of you here!), during this experience it felt like my spine had dissolved to be replaced by a light-filled serpent. I was left astounded, uplifted and more than a little confused. Given that I was in the middle of a silent retreat, I couldn't even talk to anyone about what I had experienced.

It felt like all the vertebrae in my spine had dissolved at once, to be replaced with an energy much like an electric current. Even more bizarre was the fact that this energy surge was joined by an unshakable vision of a cobra-like snake replacing my spinal column.

Seeking answers, the day I left the meditation retreat I went straight to an Internet café. Within a few minutes I'd discovered that Hindu mythology describes the "serpent power" that lies coiled at the base of the spine as a kind of universal energy. Reportedly, this energy is awakened in deep meditation or enlightenment.

However, let me offer a word of caution before your expectations are set on a one-way ticket to *nirvana*. If, like many of us, you're the kind of person who never switches off, who even on holiday has the day scheduled from dawn till dusk, the mind experience that can accompany fasting may pass you by altogether. **If you want to know yourself better, fasting in a gentle, supportive and quiet environment can help you accomplish a gentle re-boot both physically and mentally, and possibly a little spiritually too.** Fasting needs some willpower in the beginning and patience as you move forward. Creating the right environment to enter the fasting state of mind, both inside and outside the body, is really helpful.

When I first started to meditate, I tried too hard. Furiously studying the science of the mind or contorting your face into Zen-like expressions won't work. **The only way to experience meditation is actually to experience it.** It can be maddening. You'll be trying to meditate for hours and then, just when you're ready to give up, you might get a flash of something akin to what you were aiming for. Yet, in that momentary shift you might see how you could choose to do a few things differently, or how some really small things have a huge impact on you, and how easy it would be to make a few minor changes. Many great thinkers have talked about breakthroughs and inspiration. The most famous of all was probably Albert Einstein, who said that **no problem can be solved from the same level of consciousness that created it.**

So, if you do manage to get your mind to stop its usual chatter through meditation, try asking yourself a question when all is calm. For example, **if you always react to something uncomfortable by quashing the emotion with food, then meditation can create a gap to ask why.** Sometimes there's a clear answer to that question, and sometimes there isn't. Usually it takes a bit of time.

YOGA

Yoga is often lumped together with meditation since the kind of person who likes yoga is often into meditation, and vice versa. For people with a poor attention span, yoga can be a good way of getting into a calm state without the need ever to sit cross-legged.

There are many forms of yoga and it's a case of having a go and seeing which suits you best. Regardless of which tradition you choose, good yoga teachers can make you walk out of the class feeling a foot taller and ready to take on the world. My advice would be:

- If you're gentle by nature, try Hatha.

- If you're into precision and detail, go for Iyengar.

- If you like the spiritual side of yoga, opt for Sivananda.

- If you want yoga to help you sleep, try Yin.

- If you're fit and physical, Ashtanga or Vinyasa "flow" yoga will be more your bag.

- If you *really* want to sweat, try Bikram, or "hot yoga". It's not for the faint hearted and has some medical contra-indications, but it's considered seriously addictive by devotees.

SELF-CONTROL

If you're into popular psychology or consider yourself a "Tiger Mum" (or Dad), you might well have come across the famous longitudinal **"Stanford University Marshmallow Study"**, first started in the 1960s by Stanford psychology researcher Michael Mischel. The purpose of the original experiment was to find out at what age children develop the ability to wait for something they really want, and subsequent studies over many years tracked the effects of deferred gratification on a person's future success. Mischel's experiment went like this:

A marshmallow was offered to a number of hungry four-year-old children. If a child could resist eating the marshmallow, he or she was promised two instead of one. The scientists analyzed how long each child resisted the temptation of eating the marshmallow. It was discovered that the children who were better at resisting the allure of eating a marshmallow were the ones who distracted themselves, for example by singing songs, playing with their shoelaces or pretending the marshmallow was a cloud. Interestingly, those children that Mischel called "high-delayers" went on to achieve, among other things, higher SAT (standard assessment test) scores and had lower body-mass indexes as adults than those who were easier to tempt with the marshmallows.

As my husband keeps reminding me about the male sex, "Men are just kids with longer legs". In other words, **if you think that you've outgrown your four-year-old self, you're probably wrong**. A follow-up to Mischel's study group in 2011 showed that the high-delayers' characteristic remains for life (it's partly tied in with how our brains are configured). This is not good news for those of us who like an immediate fix and think "saving up for a rainy day" is for losers... and boring ones at that.

If you watch American TV, you most likely know that if you can get into the aforementioned Stanford University, you're one smart cookie. However, as a study led by Baba Shiv, Associate Professor of Marketing at Stanford's Graduate School of Business proved, **being smart doesn't mean you have better willpower**. In Shiv's experiment, several dozen undergraduates were divided into two groups. One group was given a two-digit number to remember, while the second group was given a seven-digit number. Then they were told to walk down the hall where they were presented with two different snack options – a slice of chocolate cake or a bowl of fruit salad. The students with seven digits to remember were nearly twice as likely to choose the cake as students given two digits. The researchers behind the study surmised that the results were because those extra numbers took up valuable space in the brain – they were a "cognitive load" – making it that much harder to resist a sweet fix.

Let's translate this into real life.

Jenny breaks up with her boyfriend. Does she:

a) Go home and make herself a nutritionally balanced meal, served with mineral water, ice and a twist of lime?

b) Ditch the diet in favour of "wine o'clock" with the girls?

Adam feels belittled by his boss. Does he:

a) Go to the gym and order carrot juice?

b) Hit the pub with his mates?

The point is, we've all been there and **we're fundamentally likely to let good intentions fall by the wayside if we're stressed or overwhelmed, no matter how smart we are.** In these types of situations it will be your friends or family that will keep you on track.

KNOW THE EFFECT OTHERS HAVE ON YOU

I guarantee that if you enter the world of fasting you'll meet **Mrs Doyle.** Mrs Doyle? For those of you who are not familiar with the Mrs Doyle archetype, she was the housekeeper in the classic Irish sitcom "Father Ted" whose famous catchphrase was, "Ahhh now, go on, go on, go on, go on" as she indulged the other characters with yet another tray bake (it would be rude not to accept). She's the kind of person (most typically female) who never takes no for an answer.

Frankly, when you begin fasting, your steely reserve and shrinking waistline are intimidating. Your new-found energy is probably annoying. There will be people who want to join in the fun and come along for the ride with you, but others, like Mrs Doyle, who cannot wait to topple you. They probably do it unconsciously, so don't give the feeders a hard time. Just be armed with your excuse ("doctor's orders" or "sorry, I'm allergic to Victoria sponge") and move on.

Then there are the **energy vampires**. Granted, it all sounds a tad melodramatic but I bet you can identify a time in your life when being around a certain person made you feel drained. If so, try to haul in your social network and remember that when you're fasting you're better off being selfish with your energy reserves. This is a *good* kind of selfish.

This isn't just about making a success of fasting though. **Who you hang out with has a very real impact on whether you gain weight or get slim.** A study published in the *New England Journal of Medicine* showed how powerful your friends are. Looking at a community of 12,067 people over a period of 32 years, researchers found that subjects were more likely to gain weight and become obese when their friends did. Where there was an especially close friendship between two people, the odds of influencing each other's bodies was even greater. If one friend became obese, the odds of the other friend doing the same nearly tripled. Luckily, if you hang out with slender people the effect is the same.

Mostly though, sabotage is of the self-inflicted kind. You know as well as I do how easily healthy intentions can be swept aside. The morning visit to the coffee shop for a caffeine fix ends up including a muffin, the one glass of wine becomes a bottle (oops, hic), and snuggling up on the sofa replaces the trip to the gym. You get the idea... so, keeping your own willpower on track is your main task.

CHOOSE YOUR ENVIRONMENT WISELY

Now back to my fasting in India story...

Up there in the Himalayas, the first meal of the day, a simple lentil dhal and vegetable curry, was served at noon. Escaping to eat something indulgent would involve an hour-long trek to a German bakery further up river or taking a rickshaw to the nearby town. If you were foolish enough to leave any of your treats lying around, the monkeys would steal them anyway. In other words, it was *really* hard to over-indulge.

Contrast this with normal life for most of us. **Food and the opportunity to eat are everywhere around us. Combine this with limited opportunities to be active day-to-day and you have what scientists call an "obesogenic" environment.** The term was first coined by researchers Boyd Swinburn and Garry Egger, of Deakin University, Australia, who describe it as:

> *"The sum of influences that the surroundings, opportunities, or conditions of life have on promoting obesity in individuals or populations."*

When you're fasting, especially for the first time, it makes sense to think about where you will be spending your time. For example, don't plan your weekly shop to coincide with the first morning you skip breakfast. If you're at work, empty your snack-box and stock up on herbal teas. For every life situation there will be a way to support it. Make it a rule to think this through before you begin.

There's another way that your state of mind can easily be sidetracked from calm and controlled to flustered and aggravated. A classic way we all fall off the wagon… yes, when you've had a bad night's sleep.

SLEEP LIKE A BABY

Well, maybe not exactly – sleeping like a baby would mean waking up every few hours – but you get my drift. **Quality sleep as opposed to an alcohol-induced comatose state is incredibly helpful.**

Not enough sleep makes you feel hungrier and fasting therefore becomes harder. Scientists have long been aware of the fact that **many hormones are affected by sleep disruption,** but it's only in the last few years that the hormones controlling appetite and weight have been scrutinized and linked together in this way.

Let me put it another way… **Even if you're strong willed, you still can't escape the fact that you really are a body-shaped bag of hormones.** Ghrelin and leptin are a true partnership in the hormone world. (As we saw on page 42, ghrelin is a substance produced by the intestinal tract that induces hunger or an appetite. Its counterpart leptin is responsible for telling your brain that you're full or satisfied, therefore meaning you stop eating, unless you're eating emotionally.)

These two counterparts should obviously be working in balance to make sure you're eating when you're hungry and stopping when you're full. Now, here's the rub… Levels of ghrelin are found to be *higher* in people who have either short or disrupted sleep patterns, compared to those who have 7–8 hours of good-quality sleep.

At a fundamental level, being awake at odd or irregular hours will fight with your body's natural biological rhythms, and many body functions, including digestion, hormones and metabolism, can be put out of kilter. Shift workers or the jet-set for whom changing time-zones is a regular occurrence face more of a challenge than those of us who just like to watch late-night TV every now and then. There's a reason why vending machines are all over airports and hospitals – **quick-fix sugars are just so much more enticing**

when you're exhausted. In other words, when sleep deprivation hits, you're less in control. Being tired can sabotage a diet or your healthy intentions and is one of the main reasons why baby weight's so hard to shift. So, if you're lucky enough to have a choice about when to go to sleep, don't be ashamed about turning in early.

Last of all, **it's not just a question of the *amount* of sleep you're getting, it's also about the *quality***. So what adversely affects this? Well, I'm afraid it's the usual culprits – too much caffeine, stress and late-night eating.

TO SLEEP, PERCHANCE TO DREAM

Don't be alarmed if your dreams become more vivid when you change your diet and begin fasting. This, too, is part of the fasting state of mind. Remember, fasting used to be used only for spiritual purposes – a kind of mind detoxification, if you will. Let your unconscious run riot. You could even try keeping a dream journal or diary if you believe that dreams can be instructive. At the very least it can be entertaining!

WHEN YOU WAKE UP

A rude awakening from a mobile phone isn't exactly in keeping with the Zen lifestyle. Keep morning routines as simple and painless as possible so that those pesky stress hormones don't kick in and encourage you to break your fast four hours early. Granted, not many of us are able to wake with the rising sun and the tweeting of songbirds, but at the very least, set your alarm to a soothing sound rather than something jarring.

SLEEP SOOTHERS

If your body is tired, it's easier to get to sleep. So, if you've reached the bedtime hour and still have bundles of energy, think about expending it in … er … fun ways. But if you prefer something less adult, a warm bath is a childhood classic that works just as well for big kids as little kids.

GET MENTALLY PREPARED

If you're limbering up for a fast and your mind could do with a bit of a warm-up too, here are some preparation steps to help you get into the right state of mind, courtesy of meditation teacher, Sandy Newbigging.

PREP STEP 1: BE WILLING TO CHANGE

Most people's comfort zones are actually pretty uncomfortable. Self-limiting beliefs, health problems and challenging life circumstances can become all too familiar, and with familiar there can be a sense of security. Be completely honest with yourself when considering these questions:

- Are you willing to draw a line in the sand and step out into unfamiliar territory?

- Are you willing to do things differently?

- Are you willing to trust the process, even if at the start, some parts may seem pointless?

- Are you willing to do whatever it takes to build momentum toward new healthier habits?

If yes, then great!

PREP STEP 2: BE CLEAR ABOUT THE RESULTS YOU WANT

You are both the architect and builder of your physical body. Every day, you spend 24 hours taking actions that determine your shape, weight and overall health. The great news is that it's up to you how you use your time and there are no limits to the incredible body you can build.

Knowing *why* you want to adopt your new fasting approach can help you remain motivated and stay the distance as you get the results you want. **When deciding what your goals are, it's highly recommended that you state them in a positive way.** For instance, instead of "no longer being fat" it's more compelling and motivational to focus on "being slim, full of energy and clear headed". Take a moment to consider what you want and why you want it, and write it down in a journal so you can refer to it in the future at times when you need a little reminder.

PREP STEP 3: BE EASY ON YOURSELF

The transition from your old ways to new healthier habits is much more likely to happen if you're easy on yourself. It's natural for human beings to move away from pain toward pleasure. If you associate your new eating habits with pain, discomfort or strict discipline, you're going to increase the likelihood of quitting before your new habits become second nature to you.

On the other hand, linking your new habits with pleasure is more pleasing to the mind and enhances your chances of success. **Set the intention to be gentle on yourself as you cultivate the changes you want.** There'll be times when you may fall off the wellness wagon. If this happens, refrain from beating yourself up. Instead, lift yourself up with encouraging thoughts. Praise yourself for wanting to improve your health and, in as gentle a way as possible, decide to dust yourself off, put the past behind you and move on with a positive mind and peaceful heart.

PREP STEP 4: SHAPE UP YOUR SELF-IMAGE

You are what you think you are and you will become what you think you will become. Your "self-image" is your opinion of yourself. Your self-image determines your life success because it a) impacts how you feel and b) shapes your life choices, which in turn accumulate to form your life circumstances. Even if you don't immediately believe it to be true, if you start to think intentionally about yourself as a more positive, confident and healthy person, you'll begin to make decisions that will create a person and life that reflects your self-image.

Ultimately, it can be your choice to shape your self-image in a way that will help you to feel worthy of health success. Let now be the time you choose to take control of the opinions you have about yourself.

PART 3

PUTTING FASTING INTO PRACTICE

- NUTRITIONAL RULES FOR FASTING
- FITNESS RULES FOR FASTING
- FASTING SAFELY

CHAPTER 8

NUTRITIONAL RULES FOR FASTING

EAT WELL

The problem with most fasting information is that it only focuses on the fasting bit, not on what you need to eat. **If you're eating fewer calories, what you do eat becomes even more important.** Why? We need nutrients for the glands and organs of the body to thrive and burn fat. Restricting nutrients by living on processed foods can deprive the body of the essential vitamins, minerals, fats and proteins it needs to maintain a healthy immune system, recover from injury or illness, keep muscles strong and maintain the metabolism. That's why this book includes these nutrition rules and practical fasting plans and recipes to help guide you.

RULE 1: ONLY EAT "REAL" FOOD

This means no fake food and no diet-drinks. If you grew up in the UK, chances are you'll have fond memories of bright orange corn snacks and fizzy drinks that turned your tongue red or blue. It's to be hoped that now you're "all grown up 'n' stuff", you eat lots of rocket and Parmesan salads, roasted artichoke and monkfish. If only that was the case for all of us. Celebrity chefs may make out that this is the norm but it just isn't. Most people still eat a diet full of processed, refined, low-fibre, nutrient-deficient foods.

Not all processed food is bad, though. In fact, some of it's great. Canned food without added sugar or salt and freshly-frozen fruit and veg are just a couple of examples of stellar staples for your larder. It's the low-calorie, low-fat, oh-so-easy snacks and meals that you need to watch out for since they're often loaded with chemicals and hidden sugars.

In many low-fat products the fat is simply replaced by processed carbohydrates in the form of sugar. Read the label of your regular low-fat treats (apart from dairy products where low fat is fine) and I'll bet you'll see words ending with "-ose". Various forms of sugar, be it sucrose, maltose, glucose, fructose, or the vaguely healthy-sounding corn syrup, are all bad news for weight gain, especially around the middle.

Heavily processed foods can also be high in chemicals. There's a real and present danger that **chemicals in the environment may have a blocking effect on hormones that control weight loss.** When the brain is affected by toxins, it's possible that hormone signalling is impaired. The reason why we're unsure as to the extent of the problem is that it's impossible to test for the thousands of chemicals that are contributing to the "cocktail" effect on the body. Err on the side of caution and control what you can. **Keep foods "real"!**

But what makes up a real food diet?

PROTEIN

Protein is made up of amino acids, often called the "building blocks of life", and we need all of them to stay alive and thrive. Proteins from animal sources – meat, dairy, fish and eggs – contain all the amino acids and are therefore classed as "complete" proteins. Soya beans also fall into this category. Once and for all, **eggs are healthy.** Eggs have had a tough time of it over the years. First the salmonella scare, then the unfair link to cholesterol. Eggs are low in saturated fat and if you eat eggs in the morning, you're less likely to feel hungry later in the day.

Vegetable sources provide incomplete proteins. If you're

vegetarian or vegan, you'll get your protein from nuts, seeds, legumes and grains but you need a good variety of these to ensure that you get the full range of essential amino acids.

TOP TIP:

- Include more beans and lentils in your meals. Examples include kidney beans, butter beans, chickpeas or red and green lentils. They're rich in protein and contain complex carbohydrates, which provide slow and sustained energy release. They also contain fibre, which may help to control your blood fats. Try adding them to stews, casseroles, soups and salads.

CARBOHYDRATES

Carbs are one of the most controversial topics in nutrition and weight loss. For years we've been told that we eat too much fat, and that saturated fat is the main cause of heart disease. But recently, some experts have challenged this view, suggesting that carbohydrate is responsible for the obesity epidemic and a whole host of diseases. Should we cut carbs, avoid fat or simply reduce our food intake and exercise more?

When the body is starved of carbohydrates it looks for energy in its glycogen stores. Water binds to every gram of glycogen so it's easy to get dramatic weight loss – the only problem is that it's mostly water weight! Along with those glycogen stores you'll begin to lose fat but *not* at a rate higher than a healthier (and easier) weight-loss method.

The truth is **there are healthy fats *and* healthy carbohydrates**. Avoiding carbs altogether is unnecessary and potentially dangerous. The key is in recognizing that not all carbs are created equal. Low-glycaemic index (GI) carbohydrates, found in fibre-rich fruits, beans, unrefined grains and vegetables, are important for good health and can actively support weight loss – for example, through reducing appetite and energy intake.

However, high-GI refined carbohydrates, such as those found in soft drinks, white bread, pastries, certain breakfast cereals and sweeteners, not only make it harder to lose weight but could damage long-term health. Studies show that eating a lot of high-GI carbohydrates can increase the risk of heart disease and Type-2 diabetes.

There's been a lot of research on low-carbohydrate diets in recent years. It was initially thought that they may damage bone and kidney health, but this doesn't seem to be the case unless you have a pre-existing kidney problem. **Low-carb diets can be effective for weight loss and also improve risk factors for heart disease and diabetes. However, they do carry risks.**

First, the low intake of fruit, vegetables and whole grains on a low-carb diet reduces the intake of certain vitamins and minerals, notably folate, which is vital for women who may become pregnant. Second, cutting out unrefined carbohydrates dramatically reduces the amount of fibre in the diet, which leads to constipation and changes the balance of gut bacteria. In the long term, this may increase the risk of colorectal cancer. **Finally, eating a low-carb diet based on animal protein has been associated with a significantly higher risk of mortality**. High levels of meat and dairy create substances called prostaglandins, which are inflammatory. Inflammation is bad news for the body. **Side-effects of a very low-carb diet can include bad breath, hair loss, mood swings, constipation and fatigue.** In my opinion, this is too high a price to pay when weight loss can be achieved just as quickly without the side-effects.

For this reason, while I'd never recommend cutting out carbohydrates as a food group, **my recipes focus on unrefined, low-GI carbs from whole foods rather than refined, high-GI carbs.** As well as improving health, low-GI carbs release glucose into the bloodstream more slowly, which leads to a more sustained energy release, rather than the peaks and crashes you tend to experience if you eat a lot of high-GI carbs.

TOP TIP:

- Eat bulky carbs to become slim. When you choose "big" foods like fruits, vegetables, salads and soups, which are bulked up by fibre and water, you're eating a lot of food that fills you up, but not a lot of calories.

FAT

Since fat is the greatest source of calories, eating less of it can help you to lose weight. However, fat is actually a vital nutrient and is an important part of your diet because it supplies the *essential fatty acids* needed for vitamin absorption, healthy skin, growth and the regulation of bodily functions. In fact, **eating too little fat can actually cause a number of health problems.**

The right kinds of fat, in the right amounts, can also help you to feel fuller for longer, so **try not to think of fat as your mortal diet enemy, but rather a useful ally in the pursuit of your healthier lifestyle!** Adding a little fat to your meals helps your body absorb nutrients and enhances the flavour of your food, so recipes have been created with this in mind. Choose monounsaturated fats or oils (e.g. olive oil and rapeseed oil) as these types of fats are better for your heart. Coconut oil can be a good choice for cooking as it's heat-stable.

TOP TIPS:

- Increase essential fats – aim for at least two portions of oily fish a week. Examples include mackerel, sardines, salmon and pilchards. Oily fish contains a type of polyunsaturated fat called omega 3, which helps protect against heart disease. If you don't eat fish, use flaxseed oil in salad dressing and snack on walnuts.

- If you use butter, stick to a thin scraping on bread and just a smidgen for flavour in cooking.

- Choose lean meat and fish as low-fat alternatives to fatty meats.

- Choose lower-fat dairy foods such as skimmed or semi-skimmed milk and reduced-fat natural yogurt.

- Grill, poach, steam or oven bake instead of frying or cooking with oil or other fats.

- Watch out for creamy sauces and dressings – swap them for tomato-based sauces. Add herbs, lemon, spices and garlic to reduced-fat meals to boost flavour.

- Use cheese as a topping, not a meal – in other words, no macaroni cheese! Choose cheese with a strong flavour, such as Parmesan or goat's cheese so that you only need to use a small amount.

RULE 2: CUT OUT SUGAR

Too much sugar makes you fat and has an ageing effect on the skin. Sugar links with collagen and elastin and reduces the elasticity of the skin, making you look older than your years. The recipes I provide use low-sugar fruits to add a little sweetness – and the occasional drizzle of a natural sweetener such as honey is fine – but, in general, sugar is bad news and best avoided.

TOP TIP:

- Stick to dark chocolate if you need a chocolate "fix" (which simply is the case sometimes!), as most people need less of it to feel satisfied.

RULE 3: WATCH THE ALCOHOL

Over the years the alcohol content of most drinks has gone up. A drink can now have more units than you think. A small glass of wine (175ml/5½fl oz/⅔ cup) could be as much as two units. Remember, alcohol contains empty calories so think about cutting back further if you're trying to lose weight. That's a maximum of two units of alcohol per day for a woman and three units per day for a man. For example, a single pub measure (25ml/¾fl oz) of spirit is about one unit, and a half pint of lager, ale, bitter or cider is one to one-and-a-half units.

TOP TIP:

- If you're out for the evening, try out some healthy soft drinks such as tonic with cordial, or an alcohol-free grape juice as a tasty substitute to wine. Alcohol-free beers are also becoming increasingly popular and are available in most pubs and bars.

RULE 4: EAT FRUIT, DON'T DRINK IT

If you consume around 1 litre (35fl oz/4 cups) fruit juice, remember you'll be imbibing 500 calories. That's fine if you're juice fasting, but too much if it's simply a snack. You could tuck into a baked potato with tuna and two pieces of fruit for the same amount of calories.

TOP TIPS:

- Choose herbal teas (especially green tea, which may aid fat loss).

- Feel free to have a cup or two of tea or coffee. A small amount of milk is allowed but keep it to a splash when you're fasting.

- Sip water throughout the fast, aiming for a fluid intake of around 1.2–2 litres (40–70fl oz/4¾–8 cups) a day. This will not only help to keep hunger pangs at bay, it will also keep you hydrated.

RULE 5: AVOID THE PITFALLS

TOP TIPS:

- Top up before you fast. When you first start fasting, you may feel hungry during the times when you'd normally have a meal and you may also feel slightly light-headed if you have sugary foods as your last meal. This isn't a sign that you're wasting away or entering starvation mode, and these feelings of hunger will usually subside once that usual meal time has passed. Try to get your carbohydrate intake from fruit, vegetables and whole grains and eat a good amount of protein, which will fill you up for longer. Following the fasting plans will make this as straightforward as possible.

- Stock up for quick meals. Make sure you always have ingredients in your fridge and cupboards for meals that can be put together quickly, such as stir-fries, soups and salads.

- Don't polish off the kids' plates. Eating the children's leftovers is a fast track to weight gain for parents. Put the plates straight into the sink or dishwasher when the children have finished their meal, so you won't be tempted!

- Downsize your dinner plate. Much of our hunger and satiation is psychological. If we see a huge plate only half full, we'll feel like we haven't eaten enough. But if the plate is small but completely filled, we'll subconsciously feel that we have eaten enough.

- Beware of the frappuccino effect. Black coffee only contains about 10 calories but a milky coffee can contain anything from 100 calories for a standard small cappuccino to a whopping 350+ calories for a *grande* with all the trimmings. Much like the plate size, shrink your cup size and shrink your waist line. Don't be afraid to ask for half the milk – spell it out: "Don't fill up the cup." I do it all the time and the best baristas get it right first time!

- The sandwich has become the ubiquitous carb-laden "lunch on the go". Lose the top piece of bread to cut your refined carbohydrates and instead fill up with a small bag of green salad leaves and healthy dressing.

- Don't try to change everything at once. Bad habits are hard enough to break as it is. Focus on breaking one at a time.

- If you're a parent, choose your meal skipping wisely. I've tried fasting with a toddler who doesn't understand why Mummy isn't eating and will, quite literally, shove a fistful of tuna pasta into my mouth.

- Get the portions right. If you're restricting the number of meals you're having, it makes sense that the portion sizes need to be bigger than they would be if you were eating five mini-meals a day. Use the recipe section as a guide to how big your portions should be.

CHAPTER 9

FITNESS RULES FOR FASTING

WHY EXERCISE?

That old adage, "Daily exercise maketh for a healthy life and lively mind", is all well and good, but the saboteurs of all good intentions, Temptation, Procrastination and Distraction, tend to make exercise an erratic achievement for most people.

Exercise is especially challenging if you're juggling the demands of parenthood. Even though I know I'll feel much better afterwards, some days if my husband didn't proverbially kick me out of the door with my running togs on, I myself would most likely fall victim to the three scourges. Whether it's the long-drawn-out bedtime rituals of frisky toddlers or the clearing up of spaghetti-smeared kitchen walls, parenting saps desire to do anything at all in the evening other than collapse on the sofa with a glass of wine in hand to watch the latest Scandinavian import TV series. Or maybe that's just me.

But really, do we have to exercise? It's a question I'm often asked on retreat. **Many people think that exercise is just about burning off calories, but there's so much more to it than that.** Along with helping you to achieve and maintain your ideal weight, physical activity can do the following:

- Reduce your risk of heart disease, stroke, type-2 diabetes and some cancers.

- Help keep your bones strong and healthy.

- Improve your mood, reduce feelings of stress and help you sleep better.

- Give you strength and flexibility – attributes that seem to translate as much mentally as they do physically.

I also believe that on top of all these worthy benefits, exercise adds life to your years.

Sometimes it's a simple matter of making exercise more important to you. Also, if you're paying up front for an exercise class, you may find it's harder to miss. My days are dramatically improved by 30–60 minutes of exercise, whether it's running with my dog on the beach or Pilates with the girls. Exercise provides variety, buzz, a glow, a sense of achievement and perspective, plus it helps offset any guilt about enjoying that glass of Sauvignon at the end of the day!

HOW MUCH EXERCISE DO YOU NEED?

In 2010 the World Health Organization (WHO) issued global recommendations on the amount of physical activity we need to stay healthy. They recommend that adults (aged 18–64) should build up to at least **2½ hours of moderate intensity aerobic activity, 1¼ hours of vigorous intensity activity, or a combination of the two each week.** We should also incorporate two sessions of muscle-strengthening activities, such as weight training, every week. Although **we can meet these recommendations by doing just five 30-minute workouts a week,** less than a third of British women are active enough for health. And the benefits don't stop at 30 minutes.

WHO stresses that additional benefits can be achieved if we double these minimum recommendations.

Focus is often placed on structured physical activity, such as hitting the treadmill or a spin class, but this is far from being the only factor when it comes to the calorie-burn equation. We've all heard the advice about getting off the bus a stop early, or taking the stairs instead of the lift, but in reality how useful is this? Well, just think about it... as technology progresses we're at our computers for longer and longer periods each day, we shop online rather than going to the high street, we catch up with friends over Skype or Facebook rather than meeting them in the flesh, we watch TV to relax at the end of a busy day and sometimes we're just so busy that we don't think we can allow ourselves an extra five minutes to walk rather than take the car... the thing is, if you're looking to lose weight, the total energy you burn off has to be higher than the amount you eat and **every little step helps**.

Collectively, unstructured activities are referred to as non-exercise activity *thermogenesis* **(NEAT)** and include all activity-related energy expenditure that's not purposeful exercise. NEAT is actually pretty cool since some of us actually alter NEAT levels according to what we eat without even thinking about it. In other words, **one of the secrets of the naturally slim is that they fidget and move more if they over-eat**. In fact, one of the ways I was taught to help identify different body types during my training in India was to notice how much of a fidget people were when I was consulting with them! Without fail, those who had "ants in their pants" were the naturally slender types. So if you're more of a couch potato, walking off dinner is clearly a very good idea! A basic pedometer can track how far you walk each day, and trying to beat yesterday's step count can be addictive. The next generation of activity monitors track every move you make, and some even help you to understand your sleep patterns.

WHAT COUNTS AS EXERCISE?

Physical activity doesn't just mean sweating it out at the gym – any movement that gets you slightly out of breath, feeling warm and a little bit sweaty, and that makes your heart beat faster, counts (yes, I know what you're thinking and that kind of workout counts too). **You can choose from sport, active travel, structured exercise or housework.** Even small changes are beneficial and you'll get more benefit from a brisk walk every day than from dusting off your gym membership card once a month. If you've never been very active, it's not too late to start. The key to developing an active lifestyle that you can keep up long term is to **find an activity you enjoy.**

FINDING INSPIRATION

I've found that nothing works better than a bit of inspiration when it comes to changing habits. Over the last two decades, charity events such as marathons, 10km runs, cycle sportives and adventure racing have helped to motivate people to train with a goal in mind. Who would have thought that tens of thousands of women wearing sparkly bras would happily do the "Moonwalk" through the night in London and Edinburgh, kept going only by a sense of camaraderie and a shared purpose to raise money for breast cancer research?

Gyms, too, have revolutionized – it's no longer just about feeling the burn. Classes such as Zumba®, salsa and hula hooping, where having a laugh is every bit as important as burning off calories, have become part of many people's fitness regimes. "Outdoor gyms", like those run by military fitness types, have got all shapes, sizes and ages into the mud and pushing out the press-ups of a Sunday morning. For those willing to go even further, road- or mountain-biking, kitesurfing and triathlon provide accessible competitive events that you can now do much more easily at your own level.

TOP TIPS:

- Book an active holiday to get yourself started.

- Sign up for a charity run or hike.

- Achieve inner calm with yoga or sweat it out in a Bikram studio.

- If dancing's your thing, try Sh'Bam™, the latest craze to follow Zumba®.

- If you have kids, encourage them to play active games and join in too.

- Work off job frustrations with a boxing or martial arts class.

- Treat yourself to a one-to-one with a personal trainer.

- Volunteer for a local conservation project or do some heavy-duty gardening.

- Get back to what you were good at in school – badminton and netball are popular team sports that stand the test of time.

- Improve your commute to work by walking or cycling.

SIMPLE RULES FOR EXERCISE

RULE 1: TAKE THE FIRST STEP

As the saying goes, "Every journey starts with a single step". If there's anything preventing you from taking that first step, take some time to think about how you can overcome this. From there, **set yourself a realistic activity goal** for the week. Make sure you write it down and, even better, tell a loved one that you're thinking/going to do it – it makes it more real to share your conviction.

RULE 2: TAKE IT FURTHER

The next step is to **monitor your progress** – an activity diary is an ideal way to do this – and plan to add a little more each week. Keep setting new goals and challenging yourself. Variety is also vital as you can get into a rut with your exercise programme just like with anything else. Follow the lead of international sport coaches who insist on variety to keep minds fresh and stimulated, or sign up to a sport where you'll be under the watchful gaze of a coach.

RULE 3: TAKE CARE

If you're new to exercise, or haven't done any for some time, you should **always check with your doctor before starting a new exercise programme.** The benefits of activity almost always outweigh the risks, but if you have a health condition or are just starting out, your doctor will be able to advise on any activities that you should avoid or take extra care with.

RULE 4: GO FOR THE BURN

The table on page 168 shows how long it takes a person who weighs 70kg (11st) to burn 100 calories while engaging in various activities.

You'll get the best benefits from a structured exercise plan, especially if you do some of your training at a high intensity and include some weights. But if you're not quite ready for that, fitting extra movement into your day is a good way to get started. If you take the stairs instead of the lift, get off the bus or train one stop early and are generally more active without actually working out, you could lose at least 6kg (1st) in 12 months, so long as you don't eat more to compensate! If you're already exercising regularly, instead of just focusing on doing more exercise, take every opportunity to do things the active way.

When you're fasting, a great way to boost your calorie burn is to focus on increasing your NEAT. Together with the advice below on exercising, this will make sure you're doing everything you can to achieve the best shape possible.

ACTIVITY	TIME NEEDED (MINUTES)
Skipping	8
Jogging	12
Gardening (weeding)	14
Swimming (leisurely pace)	14
Cycling (light effort)	14
Scrubbing the floor (vigorous effort)	15
Vacuuming	18
Dancing	19
Playing with children	21
Walking the dog	24
Food shopping (at the supermarket)	28
Driving a car	32
Computer work	43

You might be disheartened when the running- or step-machine tells you you've burnt 87 calories when you've been sweating for at least 15 minutes. After all, it doesn't even add up to a skinny cappuccino. Don't despair! **You burn fat even after exercise** because you primarily use carbohydrate fuel during the exercise, which takes time to replace, so in the meantime, your body burns fat for energy. In other words, your metabolism is raised for a little while after your workout.

EXERCISING AND FASTING

EXERCISE AND THE 16/8 FAST

But what about exercising while fasting? As you'll know from the "Fit You and Your Life to Fasting" chapter, the 16/8 fasting pattern is often used by people who are looking to get into their best shape ever, and workouts are usually done in a fasted state.

However, it's important to remember that most of the studies on exercise while fasted were done on men, and we know that women's bodies may respond differently. This means that, **when it comes to the 16/8 fast, the rules for men and women are slightly different.**

MEN

If you regularly take part in exercise and are already quite fit, exercising in a fasted state shouldn't be a problem. As we saw earlier (see pages 95–6), the tried-and-tested method among weight-training enthusiasts is to train before the biggest meal of the day.

If you're doing a high volume of intense aerobic training, such as running, you may find it easier to mix-and-match your training times, sometimes training before eating and sometimes training after. This is especially important if you notice that you're feeling very tired when training in a fasted state, or find that you're more susceptible to illnesses such as colds.

WOMEN

As there's very little research on training while fasted in women specifically, other than the study (see page 94) which found that women's fat metabolizing enzymes increased when training *after* eating, it's more difficult to make firm recommendations on when to exercise.

If you're very active, start by timing your workouts between meals. If you're following the 16/8 fast and skipping breakfast, this means that you should exercise during the early evening, before dinner. If you're skipping dinner, a post-breakfast or pre-lunch workout is probably best.

If you only participate in light exercise such as walking, Pilates or yoga, you should be able to do this in a fasted state. You may also wish to experiment with more intense exercise when fasted – only you can know how your body responds. But if you notice symptoms such as fatigue or increased susceptibility to common bugs, this is a sign that training in a fasted state isn't for you.

Whichever method you choose, **I recommend that during the first week of the fast you limit high-intensity exercise until you see how you respond to fasting.** As they say of eating elephants, it's easy one bite at a time.

EXERCISE AND THE 5/2 FAST

If you're going to do the 5/2 fast, it's best **to avoid prolonged or hard exercise on your 500-calorie days.** However, it's fine to do this sort of exercise a couple of hours after your first meal the following day. And do make sure that if you're exercising the day before your 500-calorie day, you end the day with a proper meal.

Although you'll be going for periods of the day without food, the fasting plan (see page 180) covers all your nutritional requirements. To ensure that you're getting everything your body needs to fuel an active lifestyle, I encourage you to eat more during your eating "windows" if you feel hungry. Keep healthy snacks to hand so that you're not tempted by junk food if hunger pangs strike.

CHAPTER 10

FASTING SAFELY

By now I hope that you have an open mind to the many benefits of fasting and that you're excited about giving it a go. If you've read this book and are still trying to decide if, when, or how to give fasting a try, remember that you'll only ever truly "get it" by trying it for yourself.

Before you launch headlong into your new fasting lifestyle, here are a few words of caution. Although fasting has been around for millennia, the science on how and when to fast is in its early stages. For example, there's very little research on how fasting affects fertility.

There are some people who should avoid fasting completely, some who should seek medical advice first, and some situations where it might not be right for *you*. Fasting isn't something that you should just jump into, and it doesn't suit everyone.

WHEN NOT TO FAST

You should avoid fasting if any of the following apply:

- You are pregnant, breastfeeding, or actively trying for a baby (it's okay to fast if you're getting your body ready to conceive, but please don't consider fasting if there's any chance you could already be pregnant).

- You have ever experienced an eating disorder.

- You are underweight

You should seek medical advice first if any of the following apply:

- **You have a long-term medical condition** such as cancer, diabetes, ulcerative colitis, epilepsy, anaemia, liver, kidney or lung disease.

- **You have a condition that affects your immune system.**

- **You are on medication**, particularly medicines that control your blood sugar, blood pressure or blood lipids (cholesterol).

POSSIBLE SIDE-EFFECTS AND HOW TO MANAGE THEM

As we learnt earlier in the book, **fasting may make you feel a bit "yucky" at first**. Many juice fasters experience headaches through caffeine withdrawal, and feeling hungry is natural when you first try a fast. These effects don't usually last long, and most people find that they're outweighed by the positive effects of fasting.

More serious side-effects may include:

- Dehydration or over-hydration.

- Feeling dizzy or light-headed.

- Extreme fatigue.

- Constipation.

- Nausea or vomiting.

- Insomnia.

- Irregular periods.

Always err on the side of caution and stop the fast if you don't feel well. You can minimize the risk of some side-effects by approaching the fast safely.

TOP TIPS:
- It's really important that you follow the nutrition rules (see the "Nutritional Rules for Fasting" chapter), and make sure that you sip fluids throughout the day.

- When it comes to water, there can be "too much of a good thing" – don't guzzle gallons of water to overcome your hunger as there's a risk that you'll over-hydrate.

- Eating the right kinds of food – by that I mean "real" food not fake food – will help you to avoid light-headedness caused by temporary dips in blood sugar. Fluid and the fibre from fruit, vegetables and whole grains will help keep your bowels regular too.

- Keep a diary when you first start fasting. Noting down what and when you've eaten and any symptoms you experience, can help you tailor the fast to suit you better.

- If you experience dizziness, have a light snack or a small glass of juice and notice if it makes you feel better.

- Ongoing tiredness or conversely difficulty getting to sleep, or a dramatic change in your menstrual cycle may be signs that fasting isn't for you.

- Levels of the stress hormone cortisol do tend to rise alongside a fast, but it's thought that this only happens if the fast lasts longer than around 18 hours after stored carbohydrate in the liver has been used up. So, if you're under a lot of stress, a shorter fast may be preferable for you than a full day at a time.

- Finally, there's a lot to be said for common sense. No one knows your body better than you do. If it doesn't feel "right", listen to your body and either adjust your approach or stop. It may simply be that you need to make some more general improvements to your eating habits before your body's ready to try fasting. Successful fasting takes some trial and error – it's not all or nothing. You may need to try and stop a few times before you find the method that suits your body. Even if fasting isn't for you, you can still use the recipes and snack ideas in this book to help you lose weight or benefit your health. Simply fit the meal frequency to your lifestyle.

- If you need extra support, visit **www.amandahamilton.com** for personalized plans and daily tips on making fasting work for you.

PART 4

FASTING PLANS AND RECIPES

FASTING PLANS

COUNTDOWN PLAN

Before starting your chosen fast, I recommend that you spend at least a week cleaning up your eating habits. This is especially important if your current diet is less than optimal. The bigger the change in your eating habits, the more likely it is that you'll experience some temporary side-effects when you first start fasting. The Countdown Plan will help you to ease your body into fasting gradually.

		BREAKFAST	MORNING SNACK	LUNCH	AFTERNOON SNACK	DINNER
COUNTDOWN DAY	DAY 1	Mango, Apple and Ginger Smoothie (p.192)	Raw power snack (p.275)	Turkey Wrap (p.231)	Protein pick-me-up (p.275)	Curried Lamb with Rice and Peas (p.253)
	DAY 2	Tomato, Pepper and Onion Scrambled Eggs (p.204)	Raw power snack (p.275)	Grilled Salmon with Harissa Quinoa (p.238)	Protein pick-me-up (p.275)	Prawn and Chickpea Balti (p.265)
	DAY 3	Nut and Seed Granola (p.201)	Raw power snack (p.275)	Split Pea Soup with Ham and Chives (p.215)		Catch-of-the-Day with Broad Beans (p.258)
	DAY 4	Creamy Sultana and Apple Muesli (p.200)		Chicken, Butternut Squash and Spinach Soup (p.213)	Protein pick-me-up (p.275)	Bean and Couscous Burgers (p.267)
	DAY 5	Antioxidant Blueberry Oatie (p.193)		Baked Fish (p.237)		Minced Beef and Mushroom Cottage Pie (p.254)
	DAY 6	Apple and Ginger Porridge (p.193)		Caribbean Vegetable Burrito (p.240)		Salmon Fish Cakes p.264)
	DAY 7			Teriyaki Beef Stir-Fry (p.233)		Chicken with Herb Gravy (p.249)

16/8 LIFESTYLE FAST

With this plan, instead of eating a morning breakfast, you break the fast around noon. All your meals are concentrated in a narrow window between 12pm and 8pm (or 1pm and 9pm). An alternative is to skip dinner and have a more substantial breakfast and morning snack. Since you're skipping a meal and a snack every day, be aware that your portions need to be slightly bigger than they would be on a typical weight-loss plan.

		BREAKFAST	MORNING SNACK	LUNCH	AFTERNOON SNACK	DINNER
FAST DAY	DAY 1			Spiced Lentil Soup (p.219) with 2 slices of rye bread	Protein pick-me-up (40g/1½oz mixed nuts) and 1 pear	Spicy Salmon with Stuffed Pepper (p.263)
	DAY 2			Sticky Chicken with Mango Couscous (p.230)	Raw power snack (1 apple and 80g/2¾oz grapes)	Lentil and Spinach Stew (p.266)
	DAY 3			Goat's Cheese, Walnut and Apple Salad (p.228) with 1 slice of rye bread	Protein-pick-me-up (125g/4½oz/½ cup fat-free Greek yogurt with berries and 1 tsp honey)	Chicken, Asparagus and Cashew Nut Stir-Fry (p.244)
	DAY 4			New Potato, Salmon and Spinach Salad (p.223), plus 25g/1oz mixed nuts and raisins	Raw power snack (hummus and vegetables)	Beef in Honey and Ginger (p.255)
	DAY 5			Butternut Squash and Miso Soup (p.218) with 2 oatcakes	Protein pick-me-up (125g/4½oz/½ cup fat-free Greek yogurt with berries and 1 tsp honey)	Mediterranean Fish with Couscous (p.260)
	DAY 6			Chicken, Mozzarella and Tomato Salad (p.220) with 2 oatcakes	Raw power snack (250ml shop-bought berry smoothie with no added sugar)	Sausage Casserole (p.252). with 1 slice of wholemeal or rye bread
	DAY 7			Kedgeree (p.236) 1 apple	Protein pick-me-up (boiled egg with vegetables)	Healthy Turkey Burger (p.250) 1 pear

5/2 LIFESTYLE FAST

On this fasting pattern, you eat normally for five days of the week, then on the remaining two days you limit your daily calorie intake to 500. To keep your eating plan as close to that followed in scientific trials, we recommend that you leave a 20-hour gap in between your last meal and lunch on the fasting days. So, for example, eat dinner at 5.30pm on Day 7 then wait until 2pm to have lunch on Day 1.

		BREAKFAST	MORNING SNACK	LUNCH	AFTERNOON SNACK	DINNER
FAST DAY	DAY 1			Large mixed salad and 1 cup of Vegetable Soup (p.216) (250 calories)		Grilled Paprika Chicken (p.246) (250 calories)
	DAY 2	Mango and Passionfruit Yoatie (p.192)	Raw power snack (p.275)	Piri-Piri Chicken (p.229)	Protein pick-me-up (p.275)	Dijon Pork Chop with Apple Cabbage (p.251)
	DAY 3	Poached Eggs (p.204) with 2 slices of rye toast	Raw power snack (p.275)	Tuna Niçoise (p.235)	Protein pick-me-up (p.275)	Green Thai Tofu Curry (p.268)
	DAY 4			1 cup of Minestrone Soup (p.217) and 1 oatcake (250 calories)		Grilled Fish with Tomatoes and Olives (p.259) (250 calories)
	DAY 5	Minted Quinoa Fruit Salad (p.195)	Raw power snack (p.275)	Prawn, Beetroot, Avocado and Mango Salad (p.225)	Protein pick-me-up (p.275)	Chicken and Red Wine Casserole (p.247)
	DAY 6	Onion Omelette with Feta and Tomatoes (p.206)	Raw power snack (p.275)	Healthy No-Bun Burgers (p.234)	Protein pick-me-up (p.275)	Vegetable Chilli (p.271)
	DAY 7	Luxury Nut Muesli with Florida Cocktail (p.198)	Raw power snack (p.275)	Asian-Style Chicken Noodle Soup (p.214)	Protein pick-me-up (p.275)	Goan Fish and Chickpea Curry (p.261)

JUICE FAST

This plan (see page 182) consists of five juices and a broth, spread evenly throughout each day. Feel free to pick and choose your juice recipes to suit your own preferences – if you want to keep shopping to a minimum then stick to a core of four or five ingredients and rotate them. However, make sure that the vegetable intake is at least equal to the fruit intake. In this plan the morning juices are a little sweeter and the afternoon juices are more vegetable based. The warm juice in the evenings is designed to taste as much as possible like pudding!

The plan is set for five days, the maximum duration I would recommend anyone should attempt on their own. However, feel free to stop after a day or two. Juice fasts are often undertaken as part of a retreat where your day would typically include yoga, walks or gentle hikes in lovely scenery, spa treatments and some educational workshops – in other words, not amidst the hustle and bustle of daily life. For this reason, most people like to try a juice fast over a weekend when they can make time and space to enjoy it.

Juices are taken at regular intervals during the day rather than sipped throughout. This is mainly for practical purposes but it's also better for your teeth. I've suggested a timetable below, but you can change it to fit your own schedule. A simple vegetable broth or miso soup is a perfect accompaniment to a juice fast – I like to sit down to a bowl of broth around 6pm during a juice day so it feels like I'm having dinner.

		9AM	11AM	1PM	3PM	6PM	9PM
FAST DAY	DAY 1	Apple Zing (p.281) Nutrient-rich apples and carrots with spicy ginger to aid digestion and circulation.	St Clement's (p.277) Citrus tickles the tastebuds and packs a powerful punch of vitamin C	Gut Soother (p.280) This blend includes pineapple and ginger to calm the digestive tract.	Green Wonder (p.285) The greens deliver B vitamins to boost energy and potassium to support cleansing. No wonder it's wonderful!	Vegetable Broth (p.272)	Warm Strawberry Spice (p.278) Pudding in a cup and an excellent source of vitamin C.
	DAY 2	Apple Tropics (p.276) A juice that's high in beta-carotene, folic acid and vitamin C.	Ultimate Liver Lover (p.279) Limonene in the lemon stimulates the gallbladder, while liver function is also helped by a hefty dose of vitamin C.	Mint Medley (p.283) Tangy and earthy, with highly concentrated nutrients including protein.	Cooling Cucumber (p.282) This refreshing combination is highly cleansing – and refreshing!	Vegetable Broth (p.272)	Warm Melon and Ginger (p.279) Ginger livens up the mild flavour of melon, an excellent source of vitamin A, known to benefit vision.
	DAY 3	Jump-Out-of-Bed Juice (p.281) Pineapple helps to reduce inflammation and congestion.	Digestion Delight (p.280) Papaya boosts digestion... and male virility.	Carrot and Celery (p.284) A delicious blend to help water retention.	Veggie Cocktail (p.285) A cleansing cocktail that delivers biotin, folic acid and manganese.	Vegetable Broth (p.272)	Warm Strawberry Spice (p.278)
	DAY 4	Grape Crunch (p.282) The sweetness of the grapes is a perfect foil for the nutrient-rich celery, a great source of natural organic sodium.	Power-Packed C (p.278) Contains three of the richest sources of vitamin C.	Veggie Apple Magic (p.282) Refreshing, alkalizing and a great source of organic sodium.	Carrot and Beetroot (p.284) Invigorating and tasty – a classic combination that delivers a mega-vitamin dose.	Vegetable Broth (p.272)	Warm Melon and Ginger (p.279)
	DAY 5	Pineappple and Pear (p.276) Pineapple is anti-inflammatory and contains bromelain, a natural digestive aid.	Florida Blue (p.277) A great source of B vitamins –perfect for stress relief!	Popeye (p.283) Spinach is a source of vitamin K and iron, giving a Popeye-style energy boost!	Golden Carrot (p.283) Carrots are full of beta-carotene.	Vegetable Broth (p.272)	Warm Strawberry Spice (p.278)

RECIPES

HOW MUCH TO COOK

Many recipes in this book serve four people, but if you are cooking only for yourself it saves time, and is also cost-effective, to cook in bulk and then freeze in individual portions.

- Chill or freeze the leftover soup or stew as soon as it has cooled down after cooking.

- All soups and stews can be kept in the fridge for up to three days, or frozen and used within three months.

- Recipes for four people can be divided into individual portions and then frozen. To freeze, pour the cooled mixture into a freezerproof container, leaving a small gap between the food and the top of the container before sealing. This will allow room for the soup or stew to expand during freezing.

- Defrost in the fridge overnight, or use the defrost setting on a microwave.

- When reheating, ensure that the food is piping hot before serving.

HOW TO JUICE

The benefits of juicing can't be had simply by slurping on smoothies or swigging from a carton of orange juice from a shop's chill cabinet.

Even "virtuous brands" often contain a slug of natural sugar which is anathema to healthy weight maintenance and can become problematic for dental health if consumed regularly. In fact, the average packaged fruit smoothie contains some 11g/¼oz sugar per 100ml (3½fl oz/⅓ cup) – or a staggering 22 teaspoons sugar per 1-litre (35floz/4 cups) carton. The peeling and blending process can also strip out the vitamin and fibre value of the ingredients.

Preparing fresh juices is vital in order to make a portion work its magic. To do this you need just one piece of equipment – a juicer (see below) – or a juice bar on speed dial. Many people initially think that juicing will be a real chore, but the majority are pleasantly surprised to find that it's much easier than they thought it would be.

JUICERS

Take note that a juicer is not the same as a blender or food processor, although some food processors might have a juicing attachment. A good juicer will separate the juice from the pulp, creating a smooth liquid that concentrates the nutrients, rather than simply blending it all together smoothie style.

The best-quality juicers will efficiently juice all types of fruit, but basic juicers do not handle soft fruits very well. For this reason, where softer fruits are used in the recipes, the method suggests that the firmer fruits are juiced first, then the soft fruits and the juice are added to a blender or food processor and processed until smooth. But if you have a high-quality juicer, you can juice all the ingredients together.

Centrifugal models are at the lower end of the price scale and work by grating fruits and vegetables, then whizzing them around like a washing-machine so that the juice separates from the fibrous pulp. The only real downside of this type of juicer is that it won't handle specialist ingredients such as herbs or wheatgrass, or deal well with stringy stalks. Depending on the model, these juicers sometimes struggle to produce much juice from soft fruits such as strawberries or blackberries. However, for novices they are probably a good starting point.

At the premium end of the market, good professional models offer power and precision and – crucially if you're serious about juicing – are easy to clean and re-assemble. This end of the market is dominated by **masticating (chewing) juicers**, sometimes known simply as "slow-speed" juicers because they use a slower extraction process that results in a slightly superior quality juice.

Of course, there's constant innovation. The latest of the premium masticating models now includes twin gears, bio-magnets and a three-stage juicing process. Granted, it sounds like something a mechanic in a garage would be telling you about, but I'm reliably informed that this produces a higher yield from the fruit and a higher bio-availability (absorption) of the super-nutritious portion it produces.

The "pro" juicers can handle any type of fruit, vegetable or herb that you choose to chuck in, but it usually takes longer to make the juice using this type of juicer as the ingredients fall into a narrower chute and therefore need more chopping. The best ones can even make ice cream! Some of them are a bit tricky to clean and so are frequently consigned to the back of the kitchen cupboard. If in doubt, ask for a recommendation from someone you know who has already invested.

Don't forget to clean your juicer. This is not a pleasant task if you leave it too long and allow the juice and pulp to become dry and sticky. The easiest way is to dismantle the juicer, bin (or compost) the pulp and rinse all the removable parts under running water as soon as you've finished. That way, it only takes a minute or two.

INGREDIENTS

The recipes on pages 276–85 use a combination of **fresh fruits and vegetables** to create healthy and vibrant juices, which not only deliver a dose of vital nutrients (vitamins, minerals and phytochemicals) but also provide energy from carbohydrates found in the fruit and veg.

You can add a tablespoon of **psyllium husks** to your juices to boost the fibre content, help slow down the absorption of sugars and keep you feeling fuller for longer. Psyllium husks are easy to find in health food shops and are relatively inexpensive. They come from *Plantago ovata*, a plant native to India, and are regularly used to help improve and maintain regular GI transit and the passage of toxins out of the body. (See also pages 82–3.)

It's also a good idea to add in an **omega-3 oil** supplement for its anti-inflammatory properties and to help with absorption of fat-soluble nutrients. (Many of the vitamins that are plentiful in fruit and vegetable are fat-soluble, which means they require additional fat intake to be absorbed properly.) This can either be a high-quality fish oil supplement in capsule form or a spoonful of vegetarian omega oil, which can be stirred into one or two of your juices. **For all supplements, follow pack instructions carefully. If you're on any medication, please check for contraindications or check with your doctor or healthcare practitioner before using them.**

And while we're on the subject... if you're trying a juice fast at home, you'll be surprised at how much produce you need, so take plenty of heavy-duty bags to carry or transport your ingredients back from the shops!

CHOOSING ORGANIC

Granted (or so farmers and supermarket PRs keep telling me), regulations and good practice mean that the use of toxic fertilizers is on the wane, and their malign effects over-rated. But why take the risk of contaminated produce if organic fruit and vegetables are available?

Organic fruit and vegetables are still at a premium price, although special offers or bulk buys through the major supermarkets make some organic produce more affordable. According to the Environmental Working Group in the USA, the fruit and vegetables most likely to contain pesticide residues if you don't go organic (listed in order, apples being the worst offenders) are:

1 Apples
2 Celery
3 Peppers
4 Peaches
5 Strawberries
6 Nectarines
7 Grapes
8 Spinach
9 Lettuce
10 Cucumber (not as bad if you peel the skin)
11 Blueberries
12 Kale

If you're not going to juice the skin, it's generally safe to go non-organic. The low-risk category for non-organic fruits includes pineapple, avocado, mango, kiwi, melon and grapefruit. Whether you choose organic or non-organic, it's always important to wash your fruit and vegetables thoroughly before you juice them.

MAKING THE PERFECT JUICE

Some of my favourite juice blends can be found in the fasting plan on page 282. Feel free to pick and choose juice recipes to suit your own preferences and by all means invent variations of your own, using similar ingredients. Variety is the spice of life so there really is no single "perfect" juice. I often find that the random "use-up-the-fruit-'n'-veg leftovers" juice tastes amazing – in the world of juicing, experimentation is a good thing. Seasonal berries can add fantastic flavour and colour, and herbs make a bland-tasting juice really flavoursome.

Remember that all fruit and vegetables should be peeled or washed before juicing.

If you decide you'd like to have a go at creating your own rather than following recipes, there are some tips below to help you.

TOP TIPS:

- Make life easier for yourself by choosing fruits and vegetables that have a high water content as these give the most yield. The harder fruits and vegetables like apples, carrots, beetroot, oranges, melons, celery and some leafy greens all juice extremely well. Forget about avocados and bananas which are only suitable for blending into smoothies.

- Sweet juices are a nice treat but are too high in sugar for the duration of a juice fast. The best combination is vegetable juices sweetened with some fruit.

- When you start juicing vegetables, use ones that you already enjoy and slowly introduce new ingredients. No great rocket science there, but if aversion kicks in because a celery juice churns your stomach, the juicing habit simply isn't going to stick.

- Vegetables grown underground, such as carrots, tend to be higher in sugar so balance these with some lower-sugar ingredients.

- Make no more than a quarter of your juice with dark green vegetables, otherwise you'll most likely find it unpalatable. Juicing leafy greens becomes much easier if you roll the leaves into a little ball and then feed this into the machine. Cucumber has a mild flavour and makes an excellent vegetable base.

- If you want to enjoy the benefits of a nutrient-dense green juice, add a quarter to half a lemon or lime to the juice to counter any bitterness.

- When juicing thick-skinned fruits such as oranges, lemons and grapefruits, remove the peel but retain as much as possible of the white, pithy part just below the skin as this contains valuable nutrients. Always remove large stones.

- Fresh root ginger is an excellent addition if you can tolerate it. Ginger not only gives your juice a little "kick" but researchers have found that it can lower blood pressure and improve blood lipids and blood sugar control.

- Introduce herbs such as parsley and coriander when your creative juices are flowing!

KEEPING JUICES

To maximize the benefits of fresh juices, drink them within 15 minutes or store very carefully. You can make your juice last longer by reducing the oxidation process. Put your juice in a glass jar with an airtight lid and fill it to the very top. Restrict the amount of air in the jar to the minimum as oxygen will oxidize and damage the juice.

If you're going to integrate juice fasting regularly into your routine you might want to invest in a food vacuum pump with a jar attachment. The juice can be stored in the jar and the vacuum pump can suck out the air to reduce oxygen damage. **If you're storing juice, the maximum amount of time recommended is 24 hours.**

BREAKFASTS

OAT, DATE AND BANANA SMOOTHIE

SERVES 1

15g/½oz ready-to-eat dried dates
1 small banana, cut in half
30g/1oz/heaped ¼ cup porridge oats
210ml/7½fl oz/scant 1 cup skimmed or
    semi-skimmed milk
140g/5oz/generous ½ cup reduced-fat
    natural yogurt
3 tbsp whey protein powder (optional)

1 Put the dates in a bowl, cover
    with warm water to soften or
    leave to soak in cold water for
    2–3 hours, then drain.
2 Put the drained dates and all
    the remaining ingredients in a
    blender or food processor and
    blend until smooth and creamy.
    Pour into a glass and serve
    immediately.

PEANUT BUTTER SMOOTHIE

SERVES 1

145ml/4¾fl oz/generous ½ cup
    skimmed or semi-skimmed milk
140g/5oz/generous ½ cup reduced-fat
    natural yogurt
2 tsp peanut butter (no added sugar
    or salt)
½ tsp cinnamon
1 tsp clear honey

1 Put the milk, yogurt, peanut
    butter and cinnamon in a
    blender or food processor and
    blend until smooth and creamy.
    Pour into a glass, stir in the
    honey and serve immediately.

MANGO, APPLE AND GINGER SMOOTHIE

SERVES 1

½ mango
8mm/⅜in piece of fresh root ginger,
    peeled and grated
210ml/7½fl oz/scant 1 cup apple juice
125g/4½oz/½ cup reduced-fat natural
    yogurt
35g/1¼oz/¼ cup whey protein powder
    (optional)
a little mineral water, if needed

1 Peel the mango using a vegetable
  peeler and slice the flesh off the
  large, central stone.
2 Put the mango in a blender or
  food processor. Add the apple
  juice yogurt and protein powder
  and blend until smooth and
  creamy. If the mixture is too
  thick, add a little mineral water,
  1 tablespoon at a time. Pour into
  a glass and serve immediately.

MANGO AND PASSIONFRUIT YOATIE

SERVES 1

¾ mango
1 passionfruit
50g/1¾oz/½ cup porridge oats
125ml/4fl oz/½ cup orange juice
125g/4½oz/½ cup reduced-fat natural
    yogurt
a little mineral water, if needed

1 Peel the mango using a vegetable
  peeler and slice the flesh off the
  large, central stone.
2 Put the mango in a blender
  or food processor. Cut the
  passionfruit in half and scoop
  out the pulp and seeds into
  the blender.
3 Add the oats orange juice and
  yogurt, and blend until smooth
  and creamy. If the mixture is too
  thick, add a little mineral water,
  1 tablespoon at a time. Pour into
  a glass and serve immediately.

ANTIOXIDANT BLUEBERRY OATIE

SERVES 1

320ml/11fl oz/scant 1⅓ cups skimmed
  or semi-skimmed milk
30g/1oz/¼ cup oatmeal
2 tbsp flaxseed
50g/1¾oz/⅓ cup blueberries
3 tbsp whey protein powder (optional)

1 Pour half the milk into a nonstick
   saucepan and bring to the boil
   over high heat, stirring frequently.
   Add the oatmeal and flaxseed,
   stir well and immediately turn
   the heat down to low. Cover the
   pan with a lid and cook for 15–30
   minutes, stirring occasionally,
   until cooked to your preferred
   texture – the longer the oatmeal
   is cooked, the smoother it will be.
2 Remove the pan from the heat
   and stir in the blueberries and the
   whey protein powder, if using.
   Allow the mixture to stand,
   covered, for 5–10 minutes. Stir
   again and serve with the
   remaining milk.

APPLE AND GINGER PORRIDGE

SERVES 1

55g/2oz/heaped ½ cup porridge oats
100ml/3½fl oz/generous ⅓ cup
  skimmed or semi-skimmed milk
¾ apple, cored and grated
1.5cm/⅝in piece of fresh root ginger,
  peeled and grated

1 Put the oats, milk and
   270ml/9½fl oz/generous 1 cup
   water in a nonstick saucepan.
   Bring to the boil over high heat,
   stirring frequently. Turn the heat
   down to medium and simmer for
   10 minutes, stirring frequently,
   until the oats are cooked through
   and creamy.
2 Stir in the apple and ginger and
   serve immediately.

FIG AND WALNUT PORRIDGE

SERVES 1

55g/2oz/heaped ½ cup porridge oats
100ml/3½fl oz/generous ⅓ cup
   skimmed or semi-skimmed milk
1½ ready-to-eat dried figs, chopped
15g/½oz/⅛ cup walnuts, chopped
¼ tsp freshly grated nutmeg
1½ tsp clear honey

1 Put the oats, milk and
   270ml/9½fl oz/generous 1 cup
   water in a nonstick saucepan.
   Bring to the boil over high heat,
   stirring frequently. Turn the
   heat down to medium and stir
   in the chopped figs. Simmer for
   10 minutes, stirring frequently,
   until the oats are cooked
   through and creamy.
2 Sprinkle the porridge with the
   walnuts, nutmeg and honey
   and serve immediately.

RAISIN QUINOA PORRIDGE

SERVES 1

70g/2½oz/heaped ⅓ cup quinoa
210ml/7½fl oz/generous ¾ cup orange
   juice
30g/1oz/¼ cup raisins
1 tsp cinnamon
125g/4½oz/½ cup reduced-fat natural
   yogurt, to serve

1 Put the quinoa, orange juice,
   raisins and cinnamon in a
   nonstick saucepan. Bring to
   the boil over high heat, stirring
   frequently. Turn the heat
   down to low and simmer for
   20 minutes, stirring occasionally,
   until all the liquid has been
   absorbed. Remove the pan
   from the heat and leave to
   stand, covered, for 10 minutes.
2 Serve topped with yogurt.

MINTED QUINOA FRUIT SALAD

SERVES 1

80g/2¾oz/heaped ⅓ cup quinoa

2 tbsp chopped mint leaves

125g/4½oz/½ cup reduced-fat natural
   yogurt

70ml/2¼fl oz/generous ¼ cup apple
   juice

1 orange

50g/1¾oz/⅓ cup blueberries

1 Put 200ml/7fl oz/generous ¾ cup water in a saucepan and bring to the boil over high heat. Add the quinoa, then turn the heat down to low and simmer for 15 minutes or until the quinoa is soft. Leave to cool.

2 Meanwhile, put the mint, yogurt and apple juice in a blender or food processor. Blend until smooth and creamy, then set aside.

3 Using a sharp knife, cut a thin slice of peel and pith from each end of the orange. Put cut-side down on a plate and cut off the peel and pith in strips. Remove any remaining pith. Cut out each segment leaving the membrane behind. Squeeze the remaining juice from the membrane into a bowl and reserve.

4 Put the segments in a serving bowl and pour in the reserved juice, then add the blueberries.

5 Pour the yogurt mixture over the fruit and toss to coat, then mix in the quinoa and serve.

IMMUNITY-BOOSTING FRUIT BURST

SERVES 1

¼ pineapple
50g/1¾oz/⅓ cup blueberries
½ kiwi fruit, peeled and sliced

DRESSING
160g/5¾oz/⅔ cup reduced-fat natural
   yogurt
2 tbsp finely chopped mint leaves
1 tsp clear honey
grated zest of ½ lemon

1 To make the dressing, put the yogurt in a bowl, then stir in the mint,
   honey and lemon zest.
2 Using a sharp knife, top and tail the pineapple, then stand the pineapple
   upright and cut off the skin from top to bottom. Slice the pineapple into
   rings and remove the core using an apple corer or a sharp knife.
3 Arrange the pineapple slices on a plate and fill the centre of each with
   the blueberries. Put the kiwi fruit around the outside, spoon the dressing
   on top and serve.

CITRUS SALAD WITH ALMONDS

SERVES 1

1 grapefruit

1 orange

2 satsumas

30g/1oz/⅓ cup flaked almonds

1 Using a sharp knife, cut a thin slice of peel and pith from each end of the grapefruit. Put cut-side down on a plate and cut off the peel and pith in strips. Remove any remaining pith. Cut out each segment leaving the membrane behind. Squeeze the remaining juice from the membrane into a bowl and reserve. Repeat with the other fruits.

2 Cut the fruit segments into bite-sized pieces, taking care to catch any juice. Mix the fruit and any juice together, scatter with the almonds and serve.

FRUIT SALAD WITH CRUNCHY NUTS

SERVES 1

½ orange

½ grapefruit

¼ cantaloupe melon, peeled, deseeded and chopped

50g/1¾oz/¼ cup strawberries, hulled

50g/1¾oz/⅓ cup blueberries

15g/½oz/scant ¼ cup flaked almonds

15g/½oz/⅛ cup hazelnuts, chopped

1½ tsp clear honey

1 Using a sharp knife, cut a thin slice of peel and pith from each end of the orange. Put cut-side down on a plate and cut off the peel and pith in strips. Remove any remaining pith. Cut out each segment leaving the membrane behind. Squeeze the remaining juice from the membrane into a bowl and reserve. Repeat with the grapefruit.

2 Put the citrus fruits and the reserved juice in a serving bowl and mix in the melon, strawberries and blueberries. Top with the almonds and hazelnuts, then drizzle with the honey and serve.

LUXURY NUT MUESLI WITH FLORIDA COCKTAIL

SERVES 1

30g/1oz/scant ⅓ cup porridge oats

10g/¼oz/⅛ cup flaked almonds

15g/½oz/⅛ cup walnuts

10g/¼oz/⅛ cup oat bran or wheat
  bran

½ ruby grapefruit

1 orange

80g/2¾oz/⅓ cup reduced-fat natural
  yogurt, to serve

1 Preheat the oven to 160°C/315°F/Gas 2½. Spread the oats, almonds,
   walnuts and bran evenly over a baking tray and cook in the oven for
   5 minutes.
2 Remove the tray from the oven, turn the mixture over and return to the
   oven for a further 5 minutes until crisp. Leave to cool for 10 minutes,
   then crumble into a serving bowl.
3 Using a sharp knife, cut a thin slice of peel and pith from each end of
   the grapefruit. Put cut-side down on a plate and cut off the peel and
   pith in strips. Remove any remaining pith. Cut out each segment leaving
   the membrane behind. Squeeze the remaining juice from the membrane
   into a bowl and reserve. Repeat with the orange. Mix the grapefruit and
   orange together with the reserved juice, put on top of the muesli
   mixture and serve with yogurt.

BANANA MUESLI

SERVES 1

35g/1¼oz/⅓ cup porridge oats
1½ tbsp whole spelt
1 banana, sliced

VANILLA MILK
280ml/9¾fl oz/generous 1 cup
   skimmed or semi-skimmed milk
¾ tsp vanilla extract
2½ tbsp whey protein powder
   (optional)

1 Preheat the oven to 160°C/315°F/Gas 2½. Spread the oats and spelt evenly over a baking tray and cook in the oven for 5 minutes.

2 Take the tray out of the oven, turn the mixture over and return to the oven for a further 5 minutes until crisp. Leave to cool for 10 minutes, then crumble into a serving bowl, and put the banana slices on top.

3 To make the vanilla milk, pour the milk into a blender or food processor and add the vanilla and protein powder, if using. Process until well mixed. Pour over the cereal and serve.

CREAMY SULTANA AND APPLE MUESLI

SERVES 1

40g/1½oz/heaped ⅓ cup porridge
  oats

30g/1oz/¼ cup sultanas

55ml/1¾fl oz/scant ¼ cup skimmed or
  semi-skimmed milk

90g/3¼oz/⅓ cup reduced-fat natural
  yogurt

1 tsp clear honey

½ tsp cinnamon

½ apple, cored and grated

½ pear, peeled, cored and sliced

1 Put the oats, sultanas, milk, yogurt, honey and cinnamon in a bowl. Stir well, cover with cling film and leave in the fridge for at least 20 minutes until the sultanas have softened and the oats are creamy.

2 Stir in the apple, and serve with pear slices on top.

NUT AND SEED GRANOLA

SERVES 4

100g/3½oz/1 cup porridge oats

2 tbsp clear honey

20g/¾oz/scant ¼ cup walnuts

20g/¾oz/¼ cup flaked almonds

2 tbsp pumpkin seeds

2 tbsp sesame seeds

TO SERVE

1 canteloupe melon, peeled, deseeded
    and cut into bite-sized pieces

200g/7oz/1 cup strawberries, hulled

320g/11¼oz/heaped 1¼ cups reduced-
    fat natural yogurt

1 Preheat the oven to 160°C/315°F/Gas 2½. Put the oats, honey, walnuts,
   almonds, pumpkin seeds and sesame seeds in a bowl and mix well.
   Spread the mixture evenly over a baking tray and cook in the oven for
   5 minutes.

2 Remove the tray from the oven, turn the mixture over and return to the
   oven for a further 5 minutes until crisp. Leave to cool for 10 minutes.
   Store in an airtight container until ready to serve. The leftover granola
   will keep in an airtight container for up to 1 month.

3 To serve, crumble the granola into serving bowls, top with melon and
   strawberries and spoon over the yogurt.

FRUITY GRANOLA

SERVES 4

180g/6¼oz/heaped 1¾ cups porridge
   oats
30g/1oz/⅓ cup flaked almonds
30g/1oz/¼ cup flaxseed
4 tsp clear honey
30g/1oz/scant ¼ cup dried apple
30g/1oz/scant ¼ cup dried apricot
30g/1oz/scant ¼ cup dried banana

VANILLA MILK
180ml/6fl oz/¾ cup skimmed or
   semi-skimmed milk
2 tsp vanilla extract

1 Preheat the oven to 180°C/350°F/Gas 4. Put the oats, almonds, flaxseed
   and honey in a bowl and stir well. Spread the mixture evenly over a
   baking tray and cook in the oven for 10 minutes.

2 Remove the tray from the oven, turn the mixture over and return to the
   oven for a further 5–10 minutes until golden brown. Leave to cool for
   10 minutes, then mix in the dried fruits and store in an airtight container
   until ready to serve. The leftover granola will keep in an airtight
   container for up to 1 month.

3 To make the vanilla milk, pour the milk and vanilla extract into a jug and
   stir well. Pour the vanilla milk over the granola and serve.

SPICED GRANOLA

SERVES 4

140g/5oz/1⅓ cups porridge oats
120g/4¼oz/1 cup mixed nuts
2 tsp cinnamon
juice of ½ orange

TO SERVE
320g/11¼oz/scant 1⅓ cups reduced-fat
natural yogurt
200g/7oz/1 cup strawberries, hulled

1 Preheat the oven to 180°C/350°F/Gas 4. Put the oats, nuts, cinnamon
   and orange juice in a bowl and stir well. Spread the mixture evenly over a
   baking tray and cook in the oven for 10 minutes. Remove the tray from
   the oven, turn the mixture over and return to the oven for a further 5–10
   minutes until golden brown. Leave to cool for 10 minutes. Store in an
   airtight container until ready to serve. The leftover granola will keep in
   an airtight container for up to 1 month.
2 Once cooled, crumble the granola into a serving glass and serve topped
   with the yogurt and strawberries.

POACHED EGGS

SERVES 1

2 tsp white wine vinegar

2 eggs

2 slices of rye bread, toasted, to serve

1 Fill a frying pan with water to a depth of about 4cm/1½in and bring to the boil over high heat. Turn the heat down to medium and add the vinegar. Crack the eggs into two cups or ramekins and gently tip the eggs into the water. Simmer over a gentle heat for 2–3 minutes, occasionally basting the tops of the eggs with water, until the whites are set and the yolks are runny, or cook for longer if you prefer your egg yolks well done.

2 Remove the eggs from the pan using a slotted spoon and drain on kitchen paper. Serve immediately on toasted rye bread.

TOMATO, PEPPER AND ONION SCRAMBLED EGGS

SERVES 1

2 eggs

1 tsp olive oil

½ tomato, diced

½ spring onion, white part only, thinly sliced

½ red pepper, deseeded and diced

salt and freshly ground black pepper

1 slice of toasted rye or wholemeal bread, or 2 oatcakes, to serve

1 Put the eggs in a small bowl and beat well. Season lightly with salt and pepper.

2 Heat the oil in a nonstick saucepan over a gentle heat. Pour the eggs into the pan and cook very gently, stirring constantly, for 1–2 minutes. Add the tomato, spring onion and red pepper and cook for a further 1–2 minutes until the mixture thickens into soft curds and is still slightly runny. Serve immediately with toasted bread or oatcakes.

MUSHROOM AND SPINACH SCRAMBLED EGGS

SERVES 1

2 eggs

1 tsp olive oil

80g/2¾oz mushrooms, chopped

½ spring onion, white part only, thinly sliced

1 small handful of spinach, chopped

salt and freshly ground black pepper

1 slice of toasted rye or wholemeal bread, or 2 oatcakes, to serve

1 Put the eggs in a small bowl and beat well. Season lightly with salt and pepper.

2 Heat the oil in a nonstick saucepan over medium heat. Add the mushrooms and spring onion and cook for 2–3 minutes, until beginning to soften.

3 Pour the eggs into the pan and cook very gently, stirring constantly, for 1–2 minutes. Add the spinach and cook for a further 1–2 minutes, stirring constantly, until the egg thickens into soft curds but is still slightly runny and the spinach starts to wilt. Serve immediately with toasted bread or oatcakes.

ONION OMELETTE WITH FETA AND TOMATOES

SERVES 1

1 tsp olive oil

¼ red onion, sliced

2 eggs

40g/1½oz reduced-fat feta cheese, crumbled

4 cherry tomatoes, cut in half

4 tbsp chopped parsley leaves

1 Heat the oil in a nonstick frying pan over medium heat, add the onion and cook for 2 3 minutes until golden.

2 Put the eggs in a small bowl and beat well, then pour them into the pan. As the egg begins to set, keep lifting the edges gently and tilting the pan to let the uncooked egg trickle underneath. Cook for 2–3 minutes until bubbling on top, then flip the omelette over and cook for a further 2–3 minutes until just set.

3 Slide the omelette on to a plate, top with the feta cheese and tomatoes, sprinkle with parsley and serve immediately.

THAI-STYLE MUSHROOM OMELETTE

SERVES 1

2 tsp olive oil

¼ garlic clove, crushed

¼ tsp chilli flakes

1 spring onion, white part only, sliced

30g/1oz/⅓ cup bean sprouts

90g/3¼oz button mushrooms, sliced

50g/1¾oz oyster mushrooms, sliced

1 tbsp tamari soy sauce

2 eggs

salt and freshly ground black pepper

1 Heat half the oil in a nonstick frying pan over medium heat. Add the garlic, chilli flakes, spring onion, bean sprouts and mushrooms and fry over high heat for 2 minutes, stirring frequently. Stir in the soy sauce, then transfer the mixture to a plate and keep it warm.

2 Put the eggs in a small bowl and beat well. Season lightly with salt and pepper. Using the same frying pan, heat the remaining oil over medium heat, then pour the egg mixture into the pan. As the egg begins to set, keep lifting the edges gently and tilting the pan to let the uncooked egg trickle underneath. Cook for 2–3 minutes until bubbling on top, then flip the omelette over and cook for a further 2–3 minutes until just set.

3 Slide the omelette on to a plate and put the mushroom mixture on top. Carefully fold the omelette in half and serve immediately.

SMOKED SALMON OMELETTE

SERVES 1

1 tsp olive oil

2 eggs

1 small handful of spinach, chopped

14 chives, chopped

70g/2½oz smoked salmon, thinly
sliced

1 Heat the oil in a nonstick frying pan over medium heat. Put the eggs in
a medium bowl and beat well. Stir in the spinach and chives, then pour
the mixture into the pan. As the egg begins to set, keep lifting the edges
gently and tilting the pan to let the uncooked egg trickle underneath.
Cook for 2–3 minutes until bubbling on top, then flip the omelette over
and cook for a further 2–3 minutes until just set.

2 Slide the omelette on to a plate and put the slices of salmon on top.
Carefully fold the omelette in half and serve immediately.

BREAKFAST BURRITO

SERVES 1

2 eggs

½ red pepper, deseeded and chopped

2 tomatoes, chopped

70g/2½oz/⅓ cup tinned haricot
  beans in water (no added salt),
  drained and rinsed

¼ red chilli, deseeded and finely
  chopped

1 tsp olive oil

1 whole-wheat tortilla

1 Put the eggs in a bowl and whisk well. Add the pepper, tomatoes,
   haricot beans and chilli and mix well.
2 Preheat the grill to medium. Heat the oil in a nonstick frying pan over
   medium heat. Add the egg mixture to the frying pan and leave to cook
   for 3–4 minutes until the egg is beginning to set, then stir and leave to
   cook for a further 1–2 minutes until cooked through.
3 Put the tortilla on the grill rack and lightly toast under the preheated
   grill.
4 Spread the egg mixture evenly over the tortilla, then fold the bottom
   edge over to enclose the filling. Fold the left- and right-hand sides of
   the tortilla across the centre, leaving the top open, and serve.

FETA AND SPINACH PANCAKES

SERVES 1

30g/1oz/scant ¼ cup wholemeal flour

½ egg, beaten

30g/1oz frozen spinach, defrosted and
  drained

30g/1oz reduced-fat feta cheese,
  crumbled

1 tsp olive oil

40g/1½oz reduced-fat soft cheese

½ tomato, diced

salt and freshly ground black pepper

1 Sift the flour into a bowl, then tip in the bran left in the sieve. Add the
  egg and beat well to form a smooth batter. Mix in the spinach and feta
  cheese, and season lightly with salt and pepper.

2 Heat the oil in a nonstick frying pan over medium heat. Add enough
  batter to thinly cover the base of the frying pan. Cook until the pancake
  begins to bubble on top, then flip it over and cook for 2–3 minutes until
  golden brown on both sides. Transfer to a plate and keep the pancake
  warm while you cook the remaining batter in the same way to make
  a second pancake. Put the soft cheese and tomato in a small bowl and
  mix well.

3 Put the pancakes on a serving plate and spread the soft cheese and
  tomato mixture over the top. Serve immediately.

APPLE AND VANILLA PANCAKES

SERVES 1

80g/2¾oz/heaped ½ cup wholemeal
    flour
¾ tsp baking powder
½ egg
80ml/2½fl oz/⅓ cup skimmed or
    semi-skimmed milk
½ apple, cored and grated

½ tsp vanilla extract
1 tsp olive oil
45ml/1½fl oz/3 tbsp reduced-fat
    natural yogurt
50g/1¾oz/¼ cup strawberries, hulled
    and sliced
2 tsp clear honey

1 Sift the flour and baking powder into a bowl and tip in the bran left in
   the sieve. Mix well. Add the egg, milk, apple and vanilla extract and beat
   to make a batter.
2 Heat the oil in a frying pan over medium heat. Add tablespoonfuls of
   batter to the pan in small rounds (you may have to do this in batches)
   and cook until the pancakes begin to bubble on top, then flip them over
   and cook for 2–3 minutes until golden brown.
3 Mix the yogurt and strawberries together in another bowl. Put the
   pancakes on a plate, top with the strawberry yogurt, then drizzle with
   the honey and serve.

PEAR AND GINGER BREAKFAST MUFFINS

SERVES 4

75g/2½oz/½ cup spelt flour

1 tsp baking powder

½ tsp bicarbonate of soda

½ tsp cinnamon

½ tsp ground ginger

a pinch of freshly grated nutmeg

75g/2½oz/¾ cup porridge oats

60ml/2fl oz/¼ cup reduced-fat natural yogurt

2 eggs

110 g/3¾oz/½ cup pear purée (or baby fruit purée)

100g/3½oz/scant ½ cup clear honey

50g/1¾oz/heaped ⅓ cup raisins

¾ pear, peeled, cored and diced

1 pot of yogurt or 1 piece of fruit per person (optional), to serve

1 Preheat the oven to 190°C/375°F/Gas 5 and line four cups of a muffin tin with paper cases. Sift the flour, baking powder, bicarbonate of soda, cinnamon and ginger into a large bowl and stir in the nutmeg and oats. Make a well in the centre of the mixture and add the yogurt, eggs, pear purée and honey, then stir gently until it forms a cake-like batter. Add the raisins and pear, then stir gently to combine.

2 Divide the mixture into the paper cases and bake for 20–25 minutes until a skewer inserted into the centre of a muffin comes out clean.

3 Leave the tin to cool on a wire rack for 5 minutes before removing the muffins from the tin and serving warm. (The muffins can be made in advance and frozen, then defrosted overnight and reheated in the morning.)

4 Serve 1 muffin per person with a pot of natural yogurt or a piece of fruit, if you like.

LUNCHES

CHICKEN, BUTTERNUT SQUASH AND SPINACH SOUP

SERVES 4

4 tsp olive oil

1 red chilli, deseeded and finely
   chopped

1 onion, finely chopped

4 small garlic cloves, crushed

320g/11¼oz skinless, boneless chicken,
   diced

1 butternut squash, peeled, deseeded
   and cut into bite-sized chunks

1.25l/44fl oz/5 cups low-sodium
   vegetable stock

120g/4¼oz/scant ½ cup red lentils

4 small handfuls of spinach

2 handfuls of coriander leaves,
   chopped

½ tsp cayenne pepper, or to taste

4 slices of wholemeal bread or
   8 oatcakes, to serve

1 Heat the oil in a large nonstick saucepan over medium heat. Reserve
   a few pieces of chilli for serving, then add the remainder to the pan
   along with the onion and garlic. Cook for 10 minutes, stirring frequently,
   until golden.

2 Add the chicken and butternut squash to the pan and stir well. Turn up
   the heat to medium–high and cook for 10 minutes, stirring occasionally.

3 Pour the stock into the pan, then add the lentils. Bring to the boil over
   high heat, then reduce the heat to medium, cover with a lid and simmer
   for 15 minutes or until the chicken is cooked through and the lentils
   are soft.

4 Stir in the spinach and three-quarters of the coriander and cook for 1–2
   minutes until the spinach has wilted. Adjust the consistency of the soup
   with boiling water, if it seems too thick.

5 Season to taste with cayenne pepper, then sprinkle with the remaining
   chilli and coriander. Serve with wholemeal bread or oatcakes.

ASIAN-STYLE CHICKEN NOODLE SOUP

SERVES 4

200g/7oz dried glass noodles

4 tsp olive oil

2 garlic cloves, crushed

8cm/3¼in piece of fresh root ginger, peeled and grated

2 onions, finely chopped

2 lemongrass stalks, crushed with the side of a knife

1.25l/44fl oz/5 cups low-sodium chicken stock

650g/1lb 7oz skinless, boneless chicken, cut into thin strips

1 carrot, cut into matchsticks

1 red pepper, deseeded and cut into matchsticks

1 small handful of coriander leaves, chopped

1½ red chillies, deseeded and finely chopped

1 Put the noodles in a heatproof bowl, cover with boiling water and leave to soak for 10–15 minutes, then drain. (If you are planning to freeze the soup, soak the noodles for 8–10 minutes so that they still have plenty of "bite".)

2 Heat the oil in a nonstick saucepan over a medium–high heat. Add the garlic, ginger, onions and lemongrass and fry, stirring frequently for 3 minutes.

3 Pour the stock into the pan, then add the chicken, carrot, pepper and noodles. Bring to the boil over high heat, then turn the heat down to medium and simmer for 5 minutes or until the chicken is cooked through.

4 Remove the pan from the heat and stir in the coriander and chillies. Leave to stand for 5 minutes, then remove and discard the lemongrass. Serve.

SPLIT PEA SOUP WITH HAM AND CHIVES

SERVES 4

1 handful of chives, finely chopped

150g/5½oz/scant ⅔ cup reduced-fat
   natural yogurt

4 tsp olive oil

1 onion, chopped

2 garlic cloves, crushed

2 carrots, diced

320g/11¼oz/scant 1½ cups split peas

1.6l/56fl oz/6½ cups low-sodium
   vegetable stock

300g/10½oz lean cooked ham,
   chopped

1 Reserve a few teaspoons of chopped chives for serving, then put
   the remainder in a small bowl with the yogurt. Mix well, then cover
   with cling film and keep in the fridge until needed.

2 Heat the oil in a large nonstick saucepan over medium heat. Add
   the onion and garlic, and fry for 6 minutes or until golden, stirring
   occasionally. Add the carrots and fry for a further 5 minutes or
   until soft.

3 Add the split peas and stock, stir and bring to the boil over high
   heat. Reduce the heat to low, partially cover with a lid and simmer
   for 1 hour or until the split peas are tender.

4 Pour the soup into a blender or food processor and blend until
   smooth. Return the soup to the rinsed saucepan and reheat gently.
   Ladle into bowls and top with the ham and the chive yogurt, and
   sprinkle over the reserved chives. Serve immediately.

VEGETABLE SOUP

SERVES 4

32 asparagus spears

4 tsp olive oil or rapeseed oil

1 onion, roughly chopped

2 garlic cloves, crushed

4 carrots, chopped into bite-sized
   pieces

280g/10oz potatoes, chopped into
   bite-sized pieces

2 leeks, sliced

1.25l/44fl oz/5 cups low-sodium
   vegetable stock

185g/6½oz/¾ cup reduced-fat natural
   yogurt

4 slices of wholemeal bread or
   8 oatcakes, to serve

1 Snap off and discard any woody ends from the asparagus stalks at the point where they break easily, then chop the asparagus into bite-sized chunks. Heat the oil in a large nonstick saucepan over medium heat. Add the onion and garlic, and cook for 2 minutes, stirring occasionally.

2 Add the carrots, potatoes, leeks, asparagus and stock, and bring to the boil over high heat. Reduce the heat to low, cover the saucepan with a lid and simmer for 15 minutes or until all the vegetables are tender.

3 Stir in the yogurt and serve with wholemeal bread or oatcakes.

MINESTRONE SOUP

SERVES 4

4 tsp olive oil

2 carrots, diced

1 onion, chopped

4 celery sticks, chopped

2 garlic cloves, chopped

4 handfuls of kale, roughly chopped

1 small handful of parsley leaves, chopped

400g/14oz/2 cups tinned cannellini beans (no added salt), drained and rinsed

550g/1lb 4oz/2¼ cups tinned chopped tomatoes

650ml/22½fl oz/generous 2½ cups low-sodium vegetable stock

40g/1oz Parmesan cheese, grated

4 slices of wholemeal bread or 8 oatcakes, to serve

1 Heat the oil in a large nonstick saucepan over medium heat. Add the carrots, onion and celery and cook for 10 minutes, stirring occasionally, until soft.

2 Add the garlic, kale and half the parsley, and cook for 2–3 minutes, stirring frequently. Add the cannellini beans, tomatoes and stock. Bring to the boil over high heat, then reduce the heat to low, cover with a lid and simmer for 30 minutes.

3 Stir in the remaining parsley, sprinkle with the Parmesan and serve with wholemeal bread or oatcakes.

BUTTERNUT SQUASH AND MISO SOUP

SERVES 4

4 tsp olive oil

1 onion, finely chopped

6cm/2½in fresh root ginger, peeled
   and grated

2 garlic cloves, crushed

1.25l/44fl oz/5 cups low-sodium
   vegetable stock

1 butternut squash, peeled, deseeded
   and chopped into bite-sized chunks

100g/3½oz/½ cup tinned sweetcorn
   (no added salt or sugar), drained

140g/5oz mushrooms, cut into
   quarters

280g/10oz firm tofu, chopped into
   bite-sized chunks

6 tbsp miso

4 slices of wholemeal bread or
   8 oatcakes, to serve

1 Heat the oil in a large nonstick saucepan over medium heat. Add the
   onion, ginger and garlic and cook for 3–5 minutes, stirring occasionally,
   until golden.

2 Pour the stock into the pan and add the butternut squash, sweetcorn,
   mushrooms and tofu. Bring to the boil over high heat, then reduce the
   heat to medium, cover with a lid and simmer for 15 minutes or until the
   squash is tender. Add the miso and stir well. Serve with wholemeal
   bread or oatcakes.

SPICED LENTIL SOUP

SERVES 4

4 tsp olive oil or coconut oil

1 onion, finely chopped

2 garlic cloves, crushed

6cm/2½in piece of fresh root ginger,
   peeled and grated

1 handful of coriander leaves, chopped

2 tsp ground allspice

¼ tsp chilli powder

800ml/28fl oz/scant 3½ cups low-
   sodium vegetable stock

200g/7oz/heaped ¾ cup red lentils

1.2l/40fl oz/4¾ cups reduced-fat
   coconut milk

4 slices of wholemeal bread or
   8 oatcakes, to serve

1 Heat the oil in a large nonstick saucepan over medium heat. Add the
   onion and cook for 5 minutes, stirring occasionally, until soft, then
   add the garlic and ginger and cook for a further 4 minutes. Stir in the
   coriander, allspice and chilli and cook for a further 3 minutes, stirring
   continuously.

2 Pour the stock into the pan, then add the lentils and coconut milk.
   Bring to the boil over high heat, then reduce the heat to medium and
   simmer for 20 minutes or until the lentils are soft. If you prefer a smooth
   soup, pour the soup into a blender and blend until smooth. Serve with
   wholemeal bread or oatcakes.

CHICKEN, MOZZARELLA AND TOMATO SALAD

SERVES 1

80g/2¾oz skinless, boneless chicken
  breast
80g/2¾oz mozzarella, sliced
4 tbsp chopped basil leaves
1 handful of salad leaves
1 tomato, sliced

DRESSING
½ tbsp pesto
½ tsp olive oil

1 Preheat the grill to medium. Put the chicken on the grill rack and grill
  for 5 minutes. Turn the chicken over and grill for a further 4–5 minutes
  until cooked through. Allow to rest for 5 minutes, then cut into slices.
2 Meanwhile, put the mozzarella, basil and salad leaves in a bowl and
  gently mix together.
3 To make the dressing, put the pesto and olive oil in a small bowl and
  stir well. Drizzle the dressing over the mozzarella salad and toss lightly,
  then transfer to a serving plate. Lay the tomato slices over the top and
  finish with the chicken slices, then serve.

CHICKEN SALAD WITH APRICOT AND MINT DRESSING

SERVES 1

½ cos or romaine lettuce, chopped

¼ cucumber, chopped

1 tomato, chopped

80g/2¾oz cooked chicken breast, sliced

3 tbsp flaked almonds

DRESSING

15g/½oz sugar-free, dried unsulphured apricots

2 tbsp chopped mint leaves

grated zest of ½ orange

1 tsp clear honey

2 tsp olive oil

½ tsp wholegrain mustard

1 tbsp white wine vinegar

1   To make the dressing, put the apricots in a heatproof bowl and pour over enough boiling water to cover. Leave to soak for 10 minutes until soft, then drain.

2   Put the apricots, mint, orange zest, honey, oil, mustard and vinegar in a food processor and blend until smooth.

3   Put the lettuce, cucumber and tomato in a bowl, pour over the dressing and toss gently. Transfer to a serving plate, top with the chicken and almonds, then serve.

SMOKED MACKEREL, BEETROOT AND BEAN SALAD

SERVES 1

1 handful of baby spinach leaves

1 cooked beetroot, peeled and sliced

2 tomatoes, sliced

70g/2½oz/⅓ cup tinned haricot
  beans (no added salt), drained and
  rinsed

120g/4¼oz smoked mackerel

DRESSING

2 tbsp reduced-fat crème fraîche

2 tbsp chopped parsley leaves

juice of ¼ lemon

1 Put all the dressing ingredients in a small bowl and whisk well.

2 Put the spinach on a serving plate. Put the beetroot, tomatoes and
  beans in a bowl and toss gently. Spoon the mixture over the spinach,
  then top with the mackerel. Drizzle with the dressing and serve.

NEW POTATO, SALMON AND SPINACH SALAD

SERVES 1

165g/5¾oz new potatoes, unpeeled
2 tbsp reduced-fat crème fraîche
16 chives, finely chopped

1 handful of baby spinach leaves
110g/3¾oz tinned salmon in spring
  water, drained

1 Put the potatoes in a saucepan, cover with water and bring to the boil over high heat, then reduce the heat to medium and simmer for 15 minutes or until tender. Drain and leave to cool for 10 minutes, then cut each potato in half.
2 Put the crème fraîche and three-quarters of the chives in a large bowl and stir well.
3 Put half the spinach on a serving plate. Roughly chop the remaining spinach and add it to the bowl with the crème fraîche mixture. Add the salmon and potatoes and mix gently.
4 Spoon the mixture over the spinach, sprinkle the remaining chives over the top and serve.

SALMON AND PUY LENTIL SALAD

SERVES 1

olive oil, for greasing

165g/5¾oz skinless and boneless
   salmon fillet

200g/7oz/1 cup tinned Puy lentils
   (no added salt), drained and rinsed

juice of ½ lemon

½ garlic clove, crushed

¼ cucumber, chopped

7 cherry tomatoes, quartered

1 handful of salad leaves

salt and freshly ground black pepper

lemon wedge, to serve

DRESSING

2 tbsp reduced-fat natural yogurt

2 tbsp chopped parsley leaves

1 To make the dressing, put the yogurt and parsley in a bowl and
   stir well.

2 Preheat the grill to high and lightly oil a baking tray. Put the salmon
   on the baking tray and grill for 4 minutes on each side until cooked
   through, the flesh is opaque and the top is slightly golden; the fish
   will flake easily when a knife is inserted into it.

3 Meanwhile, put the lentils in a bowl and add the lemon juice, garlic,
   cucumber and tomatoes. Season to taste with salt and pepper and
   toss gently.

4 Flake the salmon with a fork and mix it into the lentil mixture.

5 Put the salad leaves on a serving plate, spoon the lentil mixture
   on top and pour the dressing over. Serve with a lemon wedge for
   squeezing over.

PRAWN, BEETROOT, AVOCADO AND MANGO SALAD

SERVES 1

80g/2¾oz cooked and peeled king
  prawns
½ mango
1 cooked beetroot, peeled and roughly
  chopped
4 cherry tomatoes, cut in half
1 avocado, peeled, pitted and chopped

juice of ¼ lime
1 handful of rocket
1 handful fresh coriander leaves,
  chopped
2 tbsp chopped mint leaves
freshly ground black pepper

1 Make a shallow cut down the centre of the curved backs of the prawns.
   Pull out the black vein with a cocktail stick or your fingers, then rinse the
   prawns thoroughly. Set aside.
2 Peel the mango half using a vegetable peeler and cut the flesh into slices.
3 Put the mango, beetroot, tomatoes and avocado in a serving bowl. Top
   with the prawns, drizzle the lime juice over and toss lightly. Add the
   rocket leaves, coriander and mint, then season lightly with black pepper
   and serve.

KING PRAWN COCKTAIL

SERVES 1

80g/2¾oz cooked and peeled king
 prawns
60g/2¼oz/¼ cup tinned green lentils
 (no added salt), drained and rinsed
1 handful of salad leaves
2 tomatoes, thinly sliced
¼ cucumber, thinly sliced
½ tsp paprika

SAUCE
70g/2½oz/heaped ¼ cup reduced-fat
 natural yogurt
juice of ½ lemon
1 tbsp tomato ketchup
4 tbsp chopped parsley leaves

1 Make a shallow cut down the centre of the curved backs of the prawns.
 Pull out the black vein with a cocktail stick or your fingers, then rinse
 the prawns thoroughly. Set aside.

2 To make the sauce, put the yogurt, lemon juice, tomato ketchup and
 parsley in a bowl and mix well. Add the prawns and lentils to the sauce
 and mix well.

3 Put the salad leaves in a serving bowl, then add a layer of tomatoes
 and cucumber. Add the prawn mixture and sprinkle with the paprika,
 then serve.

IRON-BOOST BEAN SALAD

SERVES 1

60g/2¼oz/¼ cup brown rice
235g/8½oz/¾ cup tinned mixed beans
(no added salt), drained and rinsed
zest of 1 lemon
juice of ½ lemon

3 tbsp chopped coriander leaves
½ tsp olive oil
1 large handful of baby spinach leaves
salt and freshly ground black pepper

1 Rinse the rice under cold running water, then put it in a saucepan and cover with cold water. Bring to the boil and simmer for 35 minutes until tender, or according to the packet instructions. Drain.

2 Meanwhile, put the beans, lemon zest and juice, coriander and olive oil in a bowl and mix well. Season lightly with salt and pepper.

3 Stir the rice into the bean mixture. (Alternatively, if you are not eating the salad straight away, leave the rice to cool, then chill it for up to 1 day until you are ready to use it. Stir it into the bean mixture just before serving.) Put the spinach on a serving plate, spoon the rice and beans on top and serve.

GOAT'S CHEESE, WALNUT AND APPLE SALAD

SERVES 1

1 large handful of baby spinach leaves

15g/½oz/⅛ cup chopped walnuts

1 small apple, cored and sliced

1 tomato, sliced

olive oil, for drizzling

balsamic vinegar, for drizzling

55g/2oz goat's cheese, thinly sliced

salt and freshly ground black pepper

1 Put the spinach, walnuts, apple and tomato in a bowl and drizzle with olive oil and balsamic vinegar.

2 Toss well and season lightly with salt and pepper. Put the goat's cheese on top of the salad and serve.

PIRI-PIRI CHICKEN

SERVES 1

140g/5oz skinless, boneless chicken
    breast

60g/2¼oz/¼ cup brown rice

½ carrot, grated

¼ courgette, grated

4 cherry tomatoes, halved

¼ red pepper, deseeded and sliced

2 tbsp reduced-fat natural yogurt

salt and freshly ground black pepper

1 handful of salad leaves, to serve

MARINADE

1½ tsp piri-piri sauce

2 tbsp chopped coriander leaves

1 To make the marinade, put the piri-piri sauce and coriander in a small
   bowl and mix well. Put the chicken in a flat, non-metallic dish and pour
   the marinade over it. Work the marinade mixture well into the flesh
   with your fingers. Cover with cling film and leave to marinate in the
   fridge for at least 30 minutes or up to 2 hours.

2 Rinse the rice under cold running water, then put it in a saucepan and
   cover with cold water. Bring to the boil and simmer for 35 minutes until
   tender, or according to the packet instructions. Drain.

3 Preheat the grill to medium. Put the marinated chicken on the grill rack
   and grill for 4–5 minutes on each side until cooked through.

4 Put the rice in a bowl, add the carrot, courgette, tomatoes and pepper
   and mix well. Season lightly with salt and pepper.

5 Put the rice mixture on a serving plate and top with the grilled chicken.
   Drizzle with the yogurt and serve with the salad leaves.

STICKY CHICKEN WITH MANGO COUSCOUS

SERVES 1

¼ mango

¼ cucumber, diced

1 tomato, chopped into small pieces

1 tsp ground cumin

1 tbsp white wine vinegar

1½ spring onions, white part only,
   thinly sliced

1 tsp wholegrain mustard

1 tsp honey

165g/5¾oz skinless, boneless chicken
   breast, cut into thin strips

60g/2¼oz/⅓ cup couscous

10g/¼oz/⅛ cup flaked almonds

1 handful of salad leaves, to serve

1 Peel the mango quarter using a vegetable peeler and cut the flesh into
   slices. Put the mango slices in a bowl and add the cucumber and tomato,
   then toss with the cumin, vinegar and spring onions.

2 Preheat the grill to medium. Put the mustard and honey in a small bowl
   and mix well. Put the chicken on a baking tray and brush with half the
   mustard mixture. Grill for 5 minutes, then turn the chicken over and
   brush with the remaining mustard mixture. Grill for a further 5 minutes
   until the chicken is cooked through.

3 Meanwhile, put the couscous in a heatproof bowl and pour over
   80ml/2½fl oz/⅓ cup boiling water. Cover and set aside for 5–10 minutes
   until the water has been absorbed. Fluff the couscous with a fork.

4 Stir the mango mixture into the couscous, spoon on to a serving plate
   and put the chicken strips on top. Sprinkle with the almonds and serve
   with salad leaves.

TURKEY WRAP

SERVES 1

½ avocado, peeled, pitted and
   chopped
1 whole-wheat tortilla
4 cherry tomatoes, roughly chopped

50g/1¾oz cooked turkey breast,
   thinly sliced
1 small handful of rocket
1 tbsp chopped basil leaves

1 Spread the avocado evenly over the tortilla, then add a layer of
tomatoes and turkey. Top with the rocket and basil.

2 Fold the bottom edge of the tortilla over to enclose the filling, then
fold the left- and right-hand sides across the centre, leaving the top
open. Serve.

TURKEY, CHILLI AND ALMOND STIR-FRY

SERVES 1

1 tsp coconut oil

100g/3½oz skinless and boneless
   turkey breast, cut into thin strips

1.5cm/⅝in piece of fresh root ginger,
   peeled and grated

1 garlic clove, chopped

3 spring onions, white part only, sliced

1 red pepper, deseeded and sliced

70g/2½oz/heaped ⅓ cup tinned
   sweetcorn (no added sugar or salt),
   drained

3 tbsp flaked almonds

½ red chilli, deseeded and chopped

1½ tbsp tamari soy sauce

1 Heat half the oil in a nonstick frying pan or wok over medium heat.
   Add the turkey and fry for 3–5 minutes, stirring frequently, until cooked.
   Remove from the pan and set aside.

2 Heat the remaining oil in the frying pan over medium heat, then add
   the ginger, garlic, spring onions, pepper, sweetcorn, almonds and chilli
   and stir-fry for 3 minutes.

3 Return the turkey to the pan and add the soy sauce and 2 tablespoons
   water. Cook until bubbling, then tip into a bowl and serve.

TERIYAKI BEEF STIR-FRY

SERVES 1

40g/1½oz/scant ¼ cup brown basmati rice

110g/3¾oz lean sirloin steak, thinly sliced

2 tbsp teriyaki sauce

1 tsp olive oil

80g/2¾oz broccoli florets, cut in half lengthways

½ carrot, thinly sliced

½ green pepper, deseeded and thinly sliced

¼ red onion, chopped

1 Rinse the rice under cold running water, then put it in a saucepan and cover with cold water. Bring to the boil, then reduce the heat to medium and simmer for 15–20 minutes until soft, or according to the packet instructions. Drain.

2 Meanwhile, put the steak and the teriyaki sauce in a bowl and toss until the meat is well coated. Cover with cling film and leave to marinate in the fridge for 10 minutes.

3 Heat the oil in a wok over medium heat and fry the steak for 1–2 minutes on each side. Add the broccoli, carrot, pepper and onion and cook for a further 2–3 minutes, or until the meat is browned on the outside but still pink in the middle and the vegetables are slightly tender. Serve hot with the rice or leave to cool and eat cold.

HEALTHY NO-BUN BURGERS

SERVES 1

200g/7oz lean minced beef
½ onion, finely chopped
1 small garlic clove, crushed
1 tbsp chopped parsley leaves
1 tbsp tomato ketchup
1 tbsp Worcestershire sauce

½ egg white
olive oil for brushing and extra for
    drizzling
6 cherry tomatoes, cut in half
1 handful of baby spinach leaves
balsamic vinegar, for drizzling

1 Put the beef in a bowl and add the onion, garlic, parsley, tomato ketchup,
   Worcestershire sauce and egg white, then mix until well combined.
   Using your hands, divide the mixture into 2 equal pieces and roll each
   one into a ball. Flatten the balls slightly to shape each one into a burger.
2 Meanwhile, preheat the grill to medium. Brush the grill rack with oil and
   cook the burgers for 5 minutes on each side or until cooked through.
3 Put the tomatoes and spinach on a plate, drizzle with oil and balsamic
   vinegar, then put the burgers on top and serve.

TUNA NIÇOISE

SERVES 1

120g/4¼oz new potatoes, unpeeled   1 egg
1 tsp olive oil, plus extra for drizzling   1 handful of green beans
165g/5¾oz fresh tuna steak   1 handful of salad leaves

1 Put the potatoes in a saucepan, cover with water and bring to the boil over high heat, then reduce the heat to medium and simmer for 15 minutes or until tender. Drain and leave to cool for 10 minutes, then cut each potato in half.

2 Heat the oil in a nonstick frying pan over medium–high heat. Add the tuna to the pan and cook for 1–2 minutes on each side until brown on the outside but slightly pink in the centre. Remove from the pan, cut into thin slices and set aside.

3 Bring two saucepans of water to the boil over high heat, then reduce the heat to medium. Add the egg (still in its shell) to one pan, and simmer gently for 10 minutes, then remove with a slotted spoon. Meanwhile, cook the beans in the other pan for 5 minutes, then drain.

4 Plunge the egg into cold water to cool it, then peel off the shell and cut the egg into quarters. Put the egg, beans, salad leaves and potatoes in a bowl, drizzle with oil and toss gently. Spoon on to a serving plate, top with the tuna slices and serve.

KEDGEREE

SERVES 1

1 egg

125g/4½oz boneless, skinless undyed smoked haddock fillets

1 tsp olive oil

¼ onion, chopped

½ tsp curry powder

60g/2¼oz/scant ⅓ cup white basmati rice

1 tbsp reduced-fat crème fraîche

2 tbsp chopped parsley leaves

freshly ground black pepper

1 Put the egg (still in its shell) in a saucepan, cover with cold water and bring to the boil over high heat. Reduce the heat to medium and simmer for 10 minutes. Remove the egg from the pan using a slotted spoon and plunge into a bowl of cold water to cool it, then peel off the shell and finely chop the egg.

2 Put the haddock fillets in a heavy-based saucepan, pour in 200ml/ 7fl oz/scant 1 cup boiling water. Bring to the boil, then reduce the heat to medium, cover with a lid and simmer gently for 10 minutes or until the fish flakes easily when a knife is inserted into it. Lift the fish out of the pan with a slotted spoon and flake the fish with a fork. Strain and reserve the cooking liquid.

3 Heat the oil in a nonstick frying pan over medium heat. Add the onion and cook gently for 2–3 minutes, stirring occasionally, until starting to turn golden. Add the curry powder and rice, and pour in 110ml/3¾fl oz/ scant ½ cup of the reserved cooking liquid. Bring to the boil, then reduce the heat to medium, cover with a lid and simmer for 15–20 minutes until the rice is soft, topping up with extra liquid if necessary.

4 Stir in the flaked fish and continue cooking, uncovered, until all the liquid has been absorbed. Remove the pan from the heat, and stir in the crème fraîche. Season lightly with black pepper, put the egg on top, then sprinkle with the parsley and serve.

BAKED FISH

SERVES 1

1 sweet potato

12 asparagus spears

2 tomatoes

1 tsp olive oil

¼ onion, chopped

¾ garlic clove, chopped

120g/4¼oz boneless, skinless white
    fish fillets (such as cod, hake or
    haddock)

salt and freshly ground black pepper

1 Preheat the oven to 200°C/400°F/Gas 6. Pierce the skin of the sweet
   potato several times with a fork, then bake for 45–60 minutes.

2 Meanwhile, put a piece of foil large enough to wrap up the fish inside
   an ovenproof dish. Snap off and discard any woody ends from the
   asparagus stalks at the point where they break easily, and set aside.

3 With a sharp knife, cut a cross in the skin of each tomato, then put them
   in a large, heatproof bowl and pour over enough boiling water to cover.
   Leave to stand for 2 minutes, then drain. Peel off and discard the skins,
   then roughly chop the flesh.

4 Heat the oil in a nonstick frying pan over medium heat. Add the onion
   and garlic and cook for 2 minutes, stirring. Add the diced tomato, then
   spoon half the tomato and onion mixture over the foil in the ovenproof
   dish. Put the fish on top and spoon the remaining tomato mixture over,
   then season to taste with pepper. Wrap the foil around the fish to make
   a loose parcel, then bake for 20–30 minutes until the fish is cooked
   through and the flesh flakes easily when a knife is inserted into it.

5 Meanwhile, put the asparagus in a steamer and steam over high heat
   for 4–5 minutes until just tender but still slightly crunchy. Drain.

6 Transfer the asparagus and the fish to a serving plate, spoon the sauce
   from the foil parcel over the fish and season lightly with salt and pepper.
   Serve with the baked sweet potato.

GRILLED SALMON WITH HARISSA QUINOA

SERVES 1

140g/5oz salmon fillet

zest and juice of ½ lime

40g/1½oz/scant ¼ cup quinoa

1 tsp olive oil, plus extra for brushing

3 spring onions, white part only, thinly
    sliced

¾ courgette, diced

1 tsp harissa paste

2 tbsp chopped coriander leaves

lime wedge, to serve

1 Put the salmon on a plate and rub the lime zest over the flesh, then
  sprinkle with half the lime juice. Cover with cling film and leave to
  marinate at room temperature for 5 minutes.

2 Put the quinoa in a sieve and rinse well under cold running water.
  Put it in a saucepan and cover with 160ml/5¼fl oz/⅔ cup boiling water.
  Bring to the boil, then reduce the heat and simmer for 15 minutes.

3 Brush the grill rack with oil and preheat the grill to medium. Put the
  salmon on the grill rack and grill for 5–6 minutes on each side or until
  cooked through and the flesh is opaque.

4 Meanwhile, heat the oil in a nonstick frying pan over medium heat.
  Add the spring onions, courgette and harissa paste, and cook for 2–3
  minutes, stirring frequently, until the vegetables start to soften.

5 Remove the pan from the heat, add the quinoa and its cooking liquid
  and toss to coat with the harissa. Cover with a lid and leave to stand
  for 5 minutes or until all the liquid has been absorbed, then fluff up
  with a fork and stir in the coriander and remaining lime juice.

6 Serve the salmon with the quinoa and a lime wedge on the side for
  squeezing over.

HALLOUMI KEBABS WITH COCONUT COUSCOUS

SERVES 1

110g/3¾oz halloumi cheese, diced

¼ courgette, diced

¼ red onion, diced

1 red pepper, deseeded and diced

1½ tsp jerk spice

55ml/1¾fl oz/scant ¼ cup reduced-fat
   coconut milk

55g/2oz/scant ⅓ cup couscous

55g/2oz/heaped ⅓ cup frozen peas

1 spring onion, white part only, thinly
   sliced

5 tbsp chopped coriander leaves

1 Soak 2 wooden skewers in cold water for 30 minutes. Put the halloumi,
   courgette, onion, pepper and jerk spice in a bowl and toss well to coat.
   Leave to marinate for 10 minutes, then thread the halloumi and
   vegetables on to the skewers.

2 Preheat the grill to medium. Put the skewers on the grill rack and grill
   for 8–10 minutes, turning regularly until lightly golden.

3 Meanwhile, put 1 tbsp water in a saucepan and add the coconut milk.
   Bring to the boil over high heat, then stir in the couscous and peas.
   Remove from the heat and cover with a lid. Leave to stand for 10
   minutes or until all the liquid has been absorbed, then fluff up the
   couscous with a fork and stir in the spring onion and coriander.

4 Remove the halloumi and vegetables from the skewers and serve on
   top of the couscous.

CARIBBEAN VEGETABLE BURRITO

SERVES 1

¼ mango

2 tbsp tinned kidney beans (no added salt), drained and rinsed

120g/4¼oz sweet potato, peeled and chopped into 1cm/½in chunks

1 tomato, chopped into 1cm/½in chunks

½ courgette, chopped into 1cm/½in chunks

1 tsp jerk spice

70ml/2¼fl oz/scant ⅓ cup reduced-fat coconut milk

1 small handful of spinach

¼ cucumber, chopped

2 whole-wheat tortillas

1 small handful of salad leaves

1 Peel the mango quarter using a vegetable peeler and cut the flesh into slices. Put the kidney beans in a frying pan and add the sweet potato, tomato, courgette, jerk spice and coconut milk. Add 70ml/2¼fl oz/scant ⅓ cup water, bring to the boil over high heat, then reduce the heat to medium and simmer for 10–15 minutes until the vegetables are cooked.

2 Add the spinach and the mango and cook for a further 3 minutes. Transfer to a bowl and leave to cool slightly, then add the chopped cucumber.

3 Lay out the tortillas and put half the salad leaves and half the kidney bean mixture on each one. Fold the bottom edge of the tortillas over to enclose the filling, then fold the left- and right-hand sides across the centre leaving the top open, and serve.

250-CALORIE LUNCHES

Try these suggestions for delicious light lunches:

- Fresh juice made with 3 carrots and 2 apples, plus 250g/9oz/1 cup reduced-fat natural yogurt.

- 500ml/17fl oz/2 cups Vegetable Soup (see page 216) and 1 large bowl of green salad, made with 1 handful of baby spinach leaves, ¼ cucumber, ¼ grated raw cabbage, ¼ grated courgette, plus ½ grated carrot and 1 chopped radish to give a splash of colour. Drizzle with 2 tsp olive oil and 2 tsp balsamic vinegar.

- 250ml/9fl oz/1 cup Spiced Lentil Soup (see page 219), served with 2 thin rice cakes plus 1 orange.

- 250ml/9fl oz/1 cup Minestrone Soup (see page 217), served with 2 oatcakes plus 1 small apple.

- 250ml/9fl oz/1 cup Chicken, Butternut Squash and Spinach Soup (see page 213), served with 2 oatcakes.

- 1 wholemeal pitta bread, 50g/1¾oz cooked chicken breast, 1 tsp reduced-fat natural yogurt, ¼ chopped apple and a few lettuce leaves.

- Sandwich made from 2 slices of wholemeal bread, 50g/1¾oz sliced chicken, 4 cherry tomatoes, 1 handful of rocket and 1 tsp wholegrain mustard.

- Sandwich made with 2 slices wholemeal bread, 50g/1¾oz sliced turkey, 1 handful of baby spinach leaves and 1 tsp Dijon mustard.

- 75g/2½oz ready-to-eat smoked mackerel, served with 1 large handful of rocket leaves and lemon juice.

- 165g/5¾oz tinned tuna in water, drained, and 1 hard-boiled egg, served on a bed of lettuce leaves with a drizzle of balsamic vinegar.

- Chopped raw vegetable crudités – for example, 1 pepper, 1 carrot and 2 celery sticks – and 3 tbsp hummus.

- 1 small baked potato with 2 tbsp hummus, served with a small green salad, consisting of 1 handful of rocket, ¼ cucumber and ¼ green pepper.

- 140g/5oz/½ cup of tinned mixed beans (no added salt), drained, served with a little chopped garlic, a squeeze of lemon juice and 30g/1oz/⅛ cup brown rice, cooked according to the packet instructions.

- Cook 150g/5½oz shelled edamame (soya) beans (can be bought frozen and defrosted) in boiling water or steam for 3–4 minutes until soft. Blitz the cooked edamame beans with 1cm/½in piece of peeled fresh root ginger and 1 tsp low-sodium soy sauce in a blender and serve with 1 handful of mixed crudités and 150g/5½oz/scant ⅔ cup reduced-fat natural yogurt.

- 2 slices of rye bread and 2 tbsp hummus.

- 2 scrambled eggs served with 1 small slice of wholemeal toast.

- Stir some lemon juice and black pepper into 50g/1¾oz/scant ¼ cup reduced-fat cottage cheese and load into a wholemeal pitta bread with 1 handful of baby spinach leaves.

- Make a Caprese Salad using 3 sliced tomatoes, 50g/1¾oz mozzarella, 1 tbsp chopped basil leaves, and salt and pepper. Drizzle with 2 tsp olive oil.

- ½ toasted bagel with 30g/1oz reduced-fat cream cheese and 50g/1¾oz grapes.

- 2 slices of wholemeal bread, thinly spread with reduced-fat spread plus 1 small banana.

DINNERS

CHICKEN, ASPARAGUS AND CASHEW NUT STIR-FRY

SERVES 1

50g/1¾oz rice noodles

14 asparagus spears

1 tsp coconut oil, rapeseed oil or
   olive oil

1 garlic clove, finely chopped

2cm/¾in piece of fresh root ginger,
   peeled and grated

1 courgette, thinly sliced

¼ red onion, thinly sliced

165g/5¾oz skinless and boneless
   chicken breast, sliced into thin strips

juice of ½ lime

3 tbsp tamari soy sauce

2 tsp clear honey

2–3 tbsp chopped coriander leaves

1 tbsp cashew nuts

1 Put the noodles in a heatproof bowl, cover with boiling water and leave
   to soak for 10–15 minutes until soft, then drain. Snap off and discard any
   woody ends from the asparagus stalks at the point where they break
   easily, then chop the asparagus into bite-sized chunks.

2 Heat the oil in a deep, nonstick frying pan or wok over medium heat.
   Add the garlic and ginger and fry for 30 seconds, then add the courgette,
   onion and asparagus. Fry, stirring constantly, for 2 minutes. Add the
   chicken and stir-fry for a further 5–6 minutes until cooked through. Stir
   in the lime juice, soy sauce and honey. Add the noodles, coriander and
   cashew nuts, then toss well and serve immediately.

CAJUN CHICKEN WITH CRUNCHY COLESLAW

SERVES 1

165g/5¾oz skinless and boneless
  chicken breast, thinly sliced
1 tsp olive oil
1 tsp paprika
2 tsp Cajun spice
lemon wedge, to serve (optional)

COLESLAW
100g/3½oz/heaped ⅓ cup reduced-
  fat natural yogurt
1 tsp wholegrain mustard
¼ onion, thinly sliced
½ carrot, grated
¼ cucumber, finely chopped
2 tomatoes, finely chopped
¼ red cabbage, thinly sliced
1 handful of parsley leaves, finely
  chopped

1 Preheat the grill to medium. Put the chicken in a bowl, then pour over
   the oil and toss to coat. Sprinkle the paprika and Cajun spice evenly over
   the chicken.
2 Put the chicken on a baking tray and grill for 7–8 minutes on each side
   until cooked through.
3 Meanwhile, make the coleslaw. Put the yogurt and mustard in a large
   bowl and stir well. Add the remaining ingredients and mix well. Serve the
   chicken and coleslaw with a lemon wedge for squeezing over, if you like.

GRILLED PAPRIKA CHICKEN
SERVES 1

140g/5oz skinless and boneless chicken
   breast

MARINADE
1 tsp olive oil
grated zest and juice of ½ lemon
½ garlic clove, finely chopped
1 tsp paprika

TO SERVE
2 tomatoes, sliced
¼ cucumber, sliced
I large handful of salad leaves
olive oil, for drizzling
balsamic vinegar, for drizzling

1 Put all the marinade ingredients in a non-metallic dish and stir well.
Add the chicken and spoon the marinade over it. Cover with cling
film and leave to marinate in the fridge for 30 minutes, spooning the
marinade over the chicken every 5–10 minutes.
2 Preheat the grill to high. Put the marinated chicken on a grill rack and
grill for 10–15 minutes or until cooked through, turning occasionally.
3 Serve the chicken with sliced tomatoes, cucumber and salad leaves,
drizzled with olive oil and balsamic vinegar.

CHICKEN AND RED WINE CASSEROLE

SERVES 4

4 tbsp wholemeal flour

480g/1lb 1oz skinless and boneless
   chicken breast, diced

4 tsp olive oil

1 onion, chopped

4 garlic cloves, finely chopped

280ml/9¾fl oz/generous 1 cup red
   wine

about 280ml/9¾fl oz/generous 1 cup
   low-sodium chicken stock

210g/7½oz button mushrooms

4 bay leaves

2 tbsp redcurrant jelly

grated zest of 2 oranges

280g/10oz/generous 1⅓ cups brown
   rice

salt and freshly ground black pepper

4 handfuls of salad leaves, to serve

1 Preheat the oven to 200°C/400°F/Gas 6. Sprinkle the flour on to a plate,
   then add the chicken and pat it in the flour to coat completely. Season
   lightly with salt and pepper.

2 Heat the oil in a nonstick frying pan. Add the onion and cook for 4–5
   minutes until the onion is starting to turn lightly golden. Add the chicken
   and cook for a further 4 minutes, then add the garlic and cook for a
   further 1 minute. Add the wine and 280ml/9¾fl oz/generous 1 cup stock,
   stir well and bring to the boil over high heat.

3 Transfer to a casserole and add the mushrooms, bay leaves, redcurrant
   jelly and orange zest. The chicken should be well covered with the liquid;
   if necessary add a little more stock. Put a lid on the casserole and cook
   in the oven for 30 minutes or until the chicken is cooked through.

4 Meanwhile, rinse the rice under cold running water, then put it in a
   saucepan and cover with cold water. Bring it to the boil then turn the
   heat down to medium and simmer for 35 minutes or until soft, or
   according to the packet instructions. Drain. Remove and discard the
   bay leaves from the casserole before serving. Serve with the rice and
   salad leaves.

MUSTARD CHICKEN AND WINTER VEGETABLE CASSEROLE

SERVES 4

4 tsp olive oil

650g/1lb 7oz skinless and boneless chicken breast, cut into bite-sized pieces

1 onion, chopped

4 celery sticks, chopped

6 carrots, diced

1 turnip, diced

1 small handful of parsley leaves, chopped

1 small handful of thyme leaves, chopped

4 bay leaves

1l/35fl oz/4 cups low-sodium chicken stock

360g/12¾oz/scant 1½ cups reduced-fat crème fraîche

2 tbsp wholegrain mustard

4 tsp cornflour

salt and freshly ground black pepper

1 Heat the oil in a nonstick saucepan. Add the chicken and onion and fry for 3 minutes. Add the celery, carrots, turnip, parsley, thyme, bay leaves and stock. Bring to the boil over high heat, then turn the heat down to medium, cover with a lid and simmer for 30 minutes.

2 Add the crème fraîche and mustard, stirring gently. Put the cornflour in a small cup, add 120–180ml/4½–6fl oz/scant ½–¾ cup cold water and stir well to make a smooth, slightly runny paste. Slowly add the cornflour paste to the pan, and cook for 2–3 minutes, stirring constantly, until the sauce is thick and creamy. Add a little more water if necessary.

3 Season to taste with salt and pepper and ladle into serving bowls.

CHICKEN WITH HERB GRAVY

SERVES 4

4 carrots, chopped

2 red onions, chopped

2 yellow peppers, deseeded and
   chopped

4 courgettes, chopped

360g/12¾oz new potatoes, cut in half

3 tsp olive oil

1 small handful of thyme leaves,
   chopped

1 small handful of rosemary leaves,
   chopped

4 skinless and boneless chicken breasts

1 tbsp cornflour

400ml/14fl oz/generous 1½ cups
   low-sodium chicken stock

salt and freshly ground black pepper

1 Preheat the oven to 200°C/400°F/Gas 6. Put the carrots, onions,
   peppers, courgettes and potatoes in a roasting tin with 2 tsp oil and toss
   so that the vegetables are lightly coated in oil. Season to taste with salt
   and pepper and sprinkle with half the thyme and rosemary. Roast the
   vegetables for 30 minutes, then turn the vegetables over and lay the
   chicken on top, then drizzle with the remaining 1 tsp oil. Return the tin
   to the oven and cook for a further 15 minutes until the chicken is cooked.

2 Meanwhile, put the cornflour in a small bowl, add 120–180ml/4½–6fl oz/
   scant ½–¾ cup cold water and stir well to make a smooth, slightly runny
   paste.

3 Put the stock and the remaining herbs in a saucepan and bring to the
   boil over high heat. Slowly add the cornflour paste, turn the heat down
   and simmer, stirring constantly, until the gravy thickens. Season the
   gravy with salt and pepper to taste, then ladle it over the chicken and
   vegetables and serve.

HEALTHY TURKEY BURGER

SERVES 1

120g/4¼oz minced turkey

2 tbsp porridge oats

1 spring onion, white part only, thinly sliced

½ egg, beaten

1 tsp mustard

1 tbsp chopped parsley leaves

olive oil, for greasing

1 wholemeal burger bun, cut in half

1 tsp mustard

1 tsp reduced-fat crème fraîche

TO SERVE

5 cherry tomatoes

¼ pepper, deseeded and sliced

1 handful of salad leaves

1 Put the mince, oats, spring onion, egg, mustard, and parsley in a bowl and mix well. Using your hands, roll the mixture into a ball, then flatten the ball and shape into a burger.

2 Preheat the grill to medium and brush the grill rack with oil. Grill the burger for 5 minutes on each side until cooked through. For the last 1 minute of cooking time, add the two halves of the burger bun to the grill rack, cut-sides up, and toast until lightly golden. Spread the bun lightly with the mustard and crème fraîche.

3 Put the burger between the two halves of the bun and serve with tomatoes, pepper and salad leaves.

DIJON PORK CHOP WITH APPLE CABBAGE

SERVES 1

1 pork loin chop, trimmed of fat

1 tsp Dijon mustard

2 tsp rapeseed oil

5mm/¼in piece of fresh root ginger,
   peeled and grated

½ tsp cinnamon

100g/3½oz red cabbage, shredded

½ green apple, peeled and grated

1 tsp maple syrup

1 tsp cider vinegar

1 Brush both sides of the chop with the mustard and set aside.

2 Heat 1 teaspoon of the oil in a nonstick saucepan over medium–low
heat. Add the ginger and cinnamon, stir for a few seconds, then add
the red cabbage, apple and maple syrup. Stir, then reduce the heat
to low. Cover with a lid and cook for 30 minutes. Add the vinegar
to the cabbage and turn the heat up to medium. Cook for a further
5 minutes until most of the liquid has evaporated.

3 Meanwhile, heat the remaining oil in a nonstick frying pan over
medium–high heat. Add the pork and fry for 5 minutes on each side
or until cooked through. Serve with the apple cabbage.

SAUSAGE CASSEROLE

SERVES 4

4 tsp olive oil

650g/1lb 7oz reduced-fat pork or beef
sausages, cut into bite-sized chunks

2 garlic cloves, finely chopped

1 onion, chopped

1 small handful of rosemary leaves,
chopped

360g/12¾oz/1⅔ cups tinned haricot
beans (no added salt), drained and
rinsed

650g/1lb 7oz/heaped 2½ cups tinned
chopped tomatoes

3 large handfuls of kale roughly
chopped

8 tbsp reduced-fat natural yogurt

freshly ground black pepper

4 slices of rye or wholemeal bread,
to serve

1 Heat the oil in a flameproof casserole over medium heat. Add the
sausages and fry for 5–6 minutes, turning regularly, until golden
brown, then add the garlic, onion and rosemary. Turn the heat down
to low, cover with a lid and cook for 15 minutes, stirring occasionally,
until the onion is soft and golden.

2 Add the beans, tomatoes and 180ml/6fl oz/¾ cup water. Bring to
the boil over high heat, then turn the heat down to low and simmer
for 20 minutes. Stir in the kale and simmer, uncovered, for a further
10 minutes. Add the yogurt and heat through.

3 Season to taste with pepper and serve with rye or wholemeal bread.

CURRIED LAMB WITH RICE AND PEAS

SERVES 4

550g/1lb 4oz lean stewing lamb, cut
   into bite-sized chunks
4 tsp coconut oil, rapeseed oil or
   olive oil
650ml/22fl oz/generous 2½ cups
   low-sodium chicken stock
200g/7oz/1 cup brown basmati rice
2 tbsp turmeric
250g/9oz/1⅔ cups fresh or frozen peas

SAUCE
6 tbsp Indian curry paste
6 tomatoes, chopped
4 garlic cloves, finely chopped
2 onions, finely chopped
1 small handful of coriander leaves,
   chopped, plus extra to serve

1 Put all the sauce ingredients in a non-metallic bowl and mix well. Add
the lamb, rubbing the sauce in well using your fingers. Cover with cling
film and leave to marinate in the fridge for at least 6 hours or overnight.

2 Heat the oil in a nonstick frying pan over medium heat. Add the lamb
and sauce, and fry for 3–4 minutes until browned, stirring occasionally,
then transfer, to a heavy-based saucepan.

3 Add the stock to the frying pan, stirring well to deglaze the juices, then
transfer enough of this liquid from the frying pan to the saucepan to just
cover the meat. Bring to the boil over high heat then turn the heat down,
cover with a lid and simmer very gently for at least 2 hours or until the
meat is tender, stirring occasionally. Add more water if necessary.

4 Meanwhile, 30 minutes before the end of cooking time, prepare the rice.
Rinse it under cold running water, then put it in a saucepan. Add the
turmeric and enough cold water to cover by 2cm/¾in. Put a lid on the
pan and bring to the boil over high heat, then turn the heat down to
medium and simmer for 20 minutes or until almost all the liquid has
been absorbed by the rice. Add the peas and heat through briefly. Turn
off the heat and leave the rice to steam for 10 minutes or until all the
liquid has evaporated. Serve the rice and curry sprinkled with coriander.

MINCED BEEF AND MUSHROOM COTTAGE PIE

SERVES 4

650g/1lb 7oz potatoes

4 tsp olive oil, plus extra for greasing

1 onion, chopped

650g/1lb 7oz lean minced beef

360g/12¾oz mushrooms, chopped

4 tbsp tomato purée

600g/1lb 5oz/2⅓ cups tinned chopped
tomatoes

4 tbsp Worcestershire sauce

salt and freshly ground black pepper

TO SERVE

4 carrots, sliced and steamed

300g/10½oz broccoli florets, steamed

1 Put the potatoes in a saucepan, cover with cold water and bring to
   the boil over high heat. Turn the heat down to medium and simmer
   for 15–20 minutes until tender, then drain, mash and leave to cool.

2 Heat the oil in a deep, nonstick frying pan over medium heat. Add
   the onion and cook for 5 minutes until soft. Add the mince and cook,
   stirring frequently, for 10 minutes until browned.

3 Add the mushrooms and cook for a further 5 minutes. Stir in the tomato
   purée, chopped tomatoes and Worcestershire sauce, and cook, stirring
   occasionally, for 20 minutes or until most of the liquid has evaporated.
   Season to taste with salt and pepper. Meanwhile, preheat the oven to
   220°C/425°F/Gas 7.

4 Spoon the mince mixture into an ovenproof dish, then top with an even
   layer of mashed potato. Cook in the centre of the oven for 20 minutes or
   until the potato begins to brown. Serve with steamed carrots and broccoli.

BEEF IN HONEY AND GINGER

SERVES 1

165g/5¾oz lean steak, such as rump,
    cut into thin strips
1 tsp coconut oil, rapeseed oil or
    olive oil
1 pak choi, quartered
1 red pepper, deseeded and sliced
100g/3½oz/heaped 1 cup bean sprouts
4 broccoli florets

4 baby corn
a handful of sugar snap peas

MARINADE
3 tsp clear honey
2cm/¾in piece of fresh root ginger,
    peeled and grated
2 tbsp tamari soy sauce

1 To make the marinade, put the honey, ginger and soy sauce in a non-metallic bowl and mix well. Add the steak and rub the marinade into it with your fingers. Cover with a lid or cling film and leave to marinate in the fridge for 30 minutes, occasionally spooning the marinade over the beef.

2 Heat the oil in a deep, nonstick frying pan or wok over medium heat. Add the beef and cook for 2–3 minutes until brown on the outside and slightly pink in the centre. Add the pak choi, pepper, bean sprouts, broccoli, baby corn, sugar snap peas and any remaining marinade. Fry, stirring constantly, for a further 2 minutes or until the beef is cooked and the vegetables are tender. Serve immediately.

BEEF AND VEGETABLE LASAGNE

SERVES 4

4 tsp olive oil

1 onion, diced

2 garlic cloves, finely chopped

400g/14oz lean minced beef

1 red pepper, deseeded and diced

2 courgettes, diced

800g/1lb 12oz/3¼ cups tinned
chopped tomatoes

2 tsp dried mixed herbs

320g/11¼oz/1¼ cups reduced-fat
cottage cheese

280ml/9¾fl oz/generous 1 cup
skimmed or semi-skimmed milk

12 no-pre-cook whole-wheat lasagne
sheets

salt and freshly ground black pepper

TO SERVE

4 tomatoes, sliced

mixed salad leaves

1 cucumber, sliced

1 Preheat the oven to 180°C/350°F/Gas 4. Heat the oil in a saucepan over
   medium heat. Add the onion and garlic and cook for 2 minutes. Add the
   minced beef, pepper and courgettes and cook for another 5 minutes until
   the mince is brown all over. Stir in the tinned tomatoes and mixed herbs,
   and season lightly with salt and pepper.

2 Put the cottage cheese and milk in a bowl and mix well. Spoon one-third
   of the mince mixture over the base of a deep, rectangular, ovenproof
   dish and lay four of the lasagne sheets on top. Cover this with one-third
   of the cottage cheese mixture. Repeat the layers of mince, lasagne and
   cottage cheese twice more. Bake for 30–40 minutes until the lasagne
   sheets are soft. Leave to stand for 5 minutes, then serve with a salad of
   tomatoes, salad leaves and cucumber.

MEATBALLS IN RED WINE AND TOMATO SAUCE

SERVES 4

320g/11¼oz lean minced beef

2 eggs, beaten

100g/3½oz/1 cup porridge oats

1 apple, grated

1 handful of oregano, chopped, or 1 tsp
   dried oregano

olive oil, for greasing

220g/7¾oz whole-wheat spaghetti

salt and freshly ground black pepper

SAUCE

4 tsp olive oil

1 onion, diced

600g/1lb 5oz/3 cups tinned chopped
   tomatoes

2 red peppers, deseeded and diced

150ml/5fl oz/scant ⅔ cup red wine

1 handful of basil leaves, chopped

1 Put the minced beef in a bowl and season lightly with salt and pepper.
   Add the eggs, oats, apple and oregano and mix everything together with
   your hands. Divide the mixture into smallish balls the size of walnuts,
   put on a plate, cover with clingfilm and put in the fridge to chill for
   30 minutes.

2 Meanwhile, to make the sauce, heat the oil in a nonstick saucepan over
   medium-low heat. Add the onion and cook gently for 8–10 minutes until
   it has softened and started to turn golden. Add the tomatoes, peppers
   and wine and simmer very gently, uncovered, for 20 minutes.

3 Preheat the grill to medium and brush the grill rack with oil. Grill the
   meatballs for 10–15 minutes, turning regularly, until browned all over and
   cooked through.

4 Remove the meatballs from the grill and add them to the sauce for the
   last 5 minutes of cooking time. Stir in the basil.

5 Bring a saucepan of water to the boil over high heat. Add the spaghetti
   and cook for 8 minutes until tender but with a little bite, or according to
   the packet instructions. Drain. Serve the spaghetti with the meatballs
   and the sauce poured over the top.

CATCH-OF-THE-DAY WITH BROAD BEANS

SERVES 1

165g/5¾oz fresh or frozen and
   defrosted broad beans
70g/2½oz/heaped ¼ cup reduced-fat
   crème fraîche
3 tbsp skimmed or semi-skimmed milk
2 tbsp chopped parsley leaves

1 tsp wholegrain mustard
olive oil, for greasing
165g/5¾oz skinless and boneless white
   fish (such as haddock, cod or hake)
salt and freshly ground black pepper
1 large handful of baby leaf spinach,
   to serve

1 Preheat the oven to 180°C/350°F/Gas 4. Put the beans, crème fraîche,
   milk, parsley and mustard in a bowl, season to taste with salt and
   pepper and mix well.
2 Brush the base of an ovenproof dish with oil. Add three-quarters of
   the bean mixture, lay the fish on top and spoon the remainder of the
   bean mixture over the fish to keep it moist. Cover loosely with foil
   and bake for 30 minutes or until the fish flakes easily when a knife is
   inserted into it.
3 Spoon the beans on to a serving plate, lay the fish on top and serve
   with baby leaf spinach.

GRILLED FISH WITH TOMATOES AND OLIVES

SERVES 1

¼ onion, finely chopped

¾ red pepper, deseeded and finely
  chopped

70ml/2¼fl oz/scant ⅓ cup low-
  sodium vegetable stock

200g/7oz/generous ¾ cup tinned
  chopped tomatoes

1 tbsp chopped oregano leaves

7 pitted black olives, quartered

olive oil, for greasing

120g/4¼oz skinless and boneless white
  fish (such as cod, hake or haddock)

salt and freshly ground black pepper

2 handfuls of green beans, steamed,
  to serve

1 Put the onion, pepper and stock in a saucepan. Bring to the boil over
   high heat, then turn the heat down to medium, cover with a lid and
   simmer for 5 minutes. Add the tomatoes, oregano and olives, and
   season to taste with salt and pepper. Bring back to the boil over high
   heat, then turn the heat down to medium and simmer for a further
   3 minutes.

2 Preheat the grill to medium–high and brush the grill rack with oil.
   Lightly season both sides of the fish with salt and pepper, then grill
   for 5 minutes on each side until slightly golden and cooked through
   and the fish flakes easily when a knife is inserted into it.

3 Transfer the fish to a serving plate, ladle the sauce over the fish and
   serve with the green beans.

MEDITERRANEAN FISH WITH COUSCOUS

SERVES 4

4 tsp olive oil

1 onion, chopped

4 celery sticks, chopped

2 garlic cloves, crushed

2 tsp chilli flakes

720g/1lb 9oz/scant 3 cups tinned
   chopped tomatoes

150ml/5fl oz/scant ⅔ cup white wine

520ml/18fl oz/generous 2 cups
   low-sodium vegetable stock

280g/10oz/1¾ cups couscous

650g/1lb 7oz white fish (such as cod,
   hake or haddock), cut into bite-sized
   chunks

TO SERVE

grated zest of 2 lemons

1 small handful of parsley leaves,
   chopped

1 Heat the oil in a nonstick frying pan over medium heat. Add the onion,
   celery, garlic and chilli flakes and fry for 10 minutes, stirring occasionally.
   Stir in the tomatoes and cook for a further 2 minutes.

2 Add the wine and stock and bring to the boil over high heat. Boil for
   2 minutes, then add the couscous. Turn the heat down to medium and
   add the fish. Cover with a lid and simmer for 5–7 minutes until the fish
   is cooked. Add more water if the mixture becomes too dry; the couscous
   should be moist and similar to a risotto in texture.

3 Serve in a bowl, sprinkled with lemon zest and parsley.

GOAN FISH AND CHICKPEA CURRY

SERVES 4

240g/8½oz/scant 1¼ cups brown rice

1 tbsp olive oil

2 onions, chopped

1½ tbsp mild Indian curry paste, or to taste

1 red pepper, deseeded and sliced

480g/1lb 1oz/2 cups tinned chickpeas (no added salt), drained and rinsed

320ml/11fl oz/scant 1⅓ cups reduced-fat coconut milk

580ml/20¼fl oz/2⅓ cups low-sodium vegetable stock

400g/14oz skinless and boneless white fish (such as cod, hake or haddock), cut into bite-sized chunks

juice of 2 lemons

1 Rinse the rice under cold running water, then put it in a saucepan and cover with cold water. Bring to the boil, then turn the heat down to medium and simmer for 35 minutes or until soft, or according to the packet instructions.

2 Meanwhile, heat the oil in a nonstick saucepan over medium heat. Add the onions and cook for 30 seconds, then turn the heat down to low. Add the curry paste and cook for 2–3 minutes, stirring constantly, to release the flavour. Stir in the pepper, chickpeas, coconut milk and stock, and bring to the boil over high heat. Add the fish, then turn down the heat and simmer for 3–4 minutes until the fish is cooked. Stir in the lemon juice. Serve the curry with the rice.

PAN-FRIED TROUT WITH LEMON YOGURT AND ASPARAGUS

SERVES 1

125g/4½oz asparagus spears, woody
   stems removed
2 tbsp reduced-fat natural yogurt
grated zest of ½ lemon
1 tsp olive oil, plus extra for drizzling
110g/3¾oz fresh trout fillet
1 handful of salad leaves
salt and freshly ground black pepper

TO SERVE
12 cherry tomatoes, cut in half
¼ red onion, sliced
2 tbsp chopped parsley leaves

1 Put the asparagus in a steamer and cook over high heat for 5 minutes or until just tender. Transfer to a bowl and leave to cool.
2 Put the yogurt and lemon zest in another bowl, season lightly with salt and pepper, and mix well.
3 Heat the oil in a nonstick frying pan over medium–high heat. Add the trout and cook for 3–4 minutes on each side until brown on the outside but slightly pink in the centre.
4 Put the asparagus and trout on a bed of salad leaves and spoon the lemony yogurt over the top. Serve with a salad of tomatoes, onion and parsley, drizzled with olive oil and seasoned with salt and pepper.

SPICY SALMON WITH STUFFED PEPPER

SERVES 1

165g/5¾oz skinless and boneless
   salmon fillet
1 tsp harissa paste
1 red pepper
olive oil, for greasing

STUFFING
60g/2¼oz reduced-fat feta cheese,
   crumbled
1 tomato, diced
½ courgette, grated
2 tbsp chopped basil leaves
salt and freshly ground pepper

1 Put the salmon in a shallow non-metallic bowl and gently rub the harissa paste all over it. Cover with cling film and leave to marinate in the fridge for at least 30 minutes or up to 2 hours, occasionally spooning the marinade over.

2 Preheat the oven to 180°C/350°F/Gas 4. Slice the top off the pepper, remove the pith and scoop out the seeds. Put the pepper on a baking tray, brush it with oil and cook in the preheated oven for 10 minutes.

3 Meanwhile, prepare the stuffing. Put all the stuffing ingredients in a bowl, season lightly with salt and pepper, and mix well. Remove the pepper from the oven and carefully spoon in the stuffing. Return the pepper to the oven and cook for a further 10–15 minutes until the pepper is tender and the stuffing is hot.

4 Preheat the grill to medium and brush the grill rack with oil. Grill the salmon for 5 minutes on each side until cooked through and the flesh is opaque and the fish flakes easily when a knife is inserted into it. Serve the salmon with the stuffed pepper.

SALMON FISH CAKES

SERVES 1

1 sweet potato, diced

3 tsp olive oil

90g/3¼oz salmon fillet

1 spring onion, white part only, sliced

2 tbsp chopped coriander leaves

50g/1¾oz/½ cup porridge oats

salt and freshly ground black pepper

TO SERVE

¼ yellow pepper, deseeded and sliced

1 handful of watercress

8 cherry tomatoes

1 Put the sweet potato in a saucepan, cover with cold water and bring to the boil over high heat. Turn the heat down and simmer for 10–15 minutes until tender. When cooked, drain, mash and leave to cool.

2 Meanwhile, heat 1 teaspoon of the oil in a nonstick frying pan over medium heat. Add the salmon and fry for 4-5 minutes on each side or until cooked though and the flesh is opaque and the fish flakes easily when a knife is inserted into it. Transfer to a large bowl and leave to cool. Flake the salmon, using a fork.

3 Put the mashed sweet potato, spring onion and coriander in the bowl with the salmon, mix well and season to taste with salt and pepper. If the mixture is very wet, add some of the oats to bind it together. Using your hands, divide the mixture into two equal pieces and roll each one into a ball. Flatten the balls slightly to shape each one into a fish cake. Put the remaining oats in another bowl and roll each fish cake lightly in the oats so that they are evenly coated and the oats are used up.

4 Heat the remaining oil in the frying pan over medium heat. Add the fish cakes to the pan and fry for 3–4 minutes on each side until golden brown. Serve with yellow pepper, watercress and cherry tomatoes.

PRAWN AND CHICKPEA BALTI

SERVES 1

55g/2oz/¼ cup brown basmati rice

1 tsp coconut oil

¼ onion, chopped

¼ green pepper, deseeded and
chopped

1 tbsp balti curry paste

110g/3¾oz/scant ½ cup tinned
chopped tomatoes

70g/2½oz/¼ cup tinned chickpeas (no
added salt), drained and rinsed

90g/3¼oz fresh or frozen raw prawns

4 tbsp chopped coriander leaves

salt and freshly ground black pepper

1 Rinse the rice under cold running water, then put it in a saucepan and
cover with cold water. Bring to the boil, then turn the heat down to
medium and simmer for 15–20 minutes until soft, or according to the
packet instructions.

2 Meanwhile, heat the oil in a deep, nonstick frying pan or wok over a
medium–high heat. Add the onion and pepper and stir-fry for 2 minutes.
Stir in the curry paste and stir-fry for a further 2 minutes.

3 Reduce the heat to medium, then add the tomatoes and chickpeas.
Continue to cook for a further 2 minutes, stirring frequently. Add the
prawns and cook for 2–3 minutes if fresh or 5 minutes if frozen, until
all the prawns have turned pink.

4 Stir in the coriander, season with a little salt and pepper and serve the
balti on top of the rice.

LENTIL AND SPINACH STEW

SERVES 4

220g/7¾oz/heaped 1 cup brown
   basmati rice
4 tsp olive oil
1 red onion, chopped
2 garlic cloves, crushed
4 tsp curry paste (optional)
400g/14oz/scant 1⅔ cups tinned
   chopped tomatoes

80ml/2½fl oz/⅓ cup low-sodium
   vegetable stock
4 tbsp chopped thyme leaves
320g/11¼oz/heaped 1¼ cups red
   lentils, rinsed and drained
320g/11¼oz frozen spinach, defrosted

1 Rinse the rice under cold running water, then put it in a saucepan and
   cover with cold water. Bring to the boil, then turn the heat down to
   medium and simmer for 15–20 minutes until soft, or according to the
   packet instructions.
2 Heat the oil in a deep, nonstick frying pan or wok over medium heat.
   Add the onion and cook for 5 minutes until soft. Add the garlic and
   cook for a further 1 minute. Stir in the curry paste, if using, and cook
   gently for a further 1 minute.
3 Stir in the tomatoes, stock, thyme and lentils. Bring to the boil over high
   heat, then turn the heat down to medium and simmer for 10 minutes.
4 Stir in the spinach and gently heat through over low heat. Serve the stew
   with the rice.

BEAN AND COUSCOUS BURGERS

SERVES 1

40g/1½oz/¼ cup couscous

2 tsp olive oil, plus extra for drizzling

¼ red onion, chopped

½ garlic clove, finely chopped

¼ red chilli, deseeded and finely
chopped

¼ tsp cumin seeds

2 tbsp chopped coriander leaves

165g/5¾oz/heaped ¾ cup tinned
cannellini beans (no added salt),
drained and rinsed

55g/2oz/heaped ¼ cup tinned red
kidney beans (no added salt),
drained and rinsed

grated zest of ¼ lemon

¼ egg, beaten

salt and freshly ground pepper

TO SERVE

¼ onion, sliced

1 tomato, sliced

1 small handful of salad leaves

juice of ½ lemon

1 Put the couscous in a heatproof bowl and add 2 tablespoons boiling
water, cover with a lid or cling film and set aside for 5–10 minutes.

2 Meanwhile, heat 1 teaspoon of the oil in a nonstick frying pan. Add the
red onion, garlic and chilli and cook for 5 minutes, then add the cumin
seeds and coriander and cook for a further 1 minute. Remove the onion
mixture from the pan and set aside to cool slightly.

3 Put the beans in a large bowl and mash well with a potato masher to
make a coarse paste. Stir in the onion mixture, couscous, lemon zest
and egg, and season lightly with salt and pepper.

4 Using your hands, roll the mixture into a ball, divide into 2 equal pieces,
then flatten and shape each one into a burger (don't worry if it feels
moist, because the egg will set). For best results, put the burgers on a
plate, cover with cling film and chill in the fridge for 2 hours.

5 Heat the remaining oil in the frying pan over medium heat. Add the
burgers and fry for 5 minutes, then carefully turn them over and fry for a
further 5 minutes on the other side until crisp and golden. Serve with
onion, tomato and salad leaves, drizzled with lemon juice and a olive oil.

GREEN THAI TOFU CURRY

SERVES 4

180g/6¼oz rice noodles

4 tsp coconut oil, rapeseed oil or
olive oil

1 red onion, chopped

2 garlic cloves, finely chopped

6cm/2½in piece of fresh root ginger,
peeled and grated

2 green chillies, deseeded and finely
chopped

650g/1lb 7oz firm tofu, cut into
2.5cm/1in cubes

875ml/30fl oz/3½ cups reduced-fat
coconut milk

2 lemongrass stalks, crushed with the
side of a knife

280g/10oz baby corn

1 red pepper, deseeded and sliced

300g/10½oz broccoli florets

4 tbsp tamari soy sauce

juice of 2 limes

1 small handful of fresh coriander,
chopped

1 Put the noodles in a heatproof bowl, cover with boiling water and leave
to soak for 10–15 minutes until soft, then drain.

2 Heat the oil in a deep, nonstick frying pan or wok over medium heat.
Add the onion, garlic, ginger and chillies and cook for 3 minutes until
soft. Add the tofu, coconut milk, lemongrass, baby corn, red pepper and
broccoli. Bring to the boil over high heat, then turn the heat down to
medium and simmer for 10 minutes. Add the noodles, soy sauce, lime
juice and coriander and simmer for a further 2 minutes, then remove the
lemongrass and discard. Serve immediately.

THAI TOFU NOODLE SOUP

SERVES 4

220g/7¾oz rice noodles

4 tsp coconut oil, rapeseed oil or
olive oil

2 red onions, sliced

4 garlic cloves, crushed

6cm/2½in piece of fresh root ginger,
peeled and grated

1 tsp chilli flakes

2 carrots, sliced

3 red peppers, deseeded and sliced

1 Chinese cabbage, sliced

560g/1lb 5oz firm tofu, cut into
bite-sized cubes

600ml/21fl oz/scant 2½ cups reduced-
fat coconut milk

1.2l/40fl oz/4¾ cups low-sodium
vegetable stock

2 handfuls of coriander leaves,
chopped

juice of 2 limes

1 Put the noodles in a heatproof bowl, cover with boiling water and
   leave to soak for 10 minutes until almost soft, then drain.

2 Heat the oil in a deep, nonstick frying pan or wok over medium heat.
   Add the onions and fry for 30 seconds, then add the garlic, ginger
   and chilli and fry, stirring constantly, for a further 30 seconds. Add
   the carrots, peppers and Chinese cabbage, and continue to stir-fry
   for a further 2–3 minutes. Add the noodles, tofu, coconut milk, stock
   and coriander. Bring to the boil over high heat, then turn the heat
   down to medium and simmer for a further 2–3 minutes until the
   noodles are cooked. Stir in the lime juice and serve.

MIDDLE-EASTERN BAKE

SERVES 4

4 tsp olive oil

1 onion, chopped

2 garlic cloves, crushed

6 carrots, diced

2 sweet potatoes, diced

320g/11¼oz/1⅓ cups tinned
  chickpeas (no added salt), drained
  and rinsed

140g/5oz/heaped ½ cup red lentils,
  rinsed and drained

4 oranges, segmented

55g/2oz/scant ⅔ cup flaked almonds

juice of 2 lemons

2 tsp ground cinnamon

2 tbsp ground cumin

1 small handful of coriander leaves,
  chopped

1 small handful of salad leaves,
  to serve

1 Preheat the oven to 200°C/400°F/Gas 6. Heat the oil in a flameproof
   casserole over medium heat. Add the onion and garlic and cook for
   3–4 minutes, stirring occasionally, until soft.

2 Add the carrots, sweet potatoes, chickpeas, lentils and 800ml/28fl oz/
   scant 3½ cups water. Bring to the boil over high heat, then turn the
   heat down to medium and cook for 10 minutes.

3 Using a sharp knife, cut a thin slice of peel and pith from each end of
   an orange. Put cut-side down on a plate and cut off the peel and pith
   in strips. Remove any remaining pith. Cut out each segment leaving the
   membrane behind. Squeeze the remaining juice from the membrane
   into a bowl and reserve. Repeat with the other oranges. Tip the almonds
   into the casserole and add the orange segments, reserved orange juice,
   lemon juice, cinnamon and cumin. Transfer to the oven and cook for
   40 minutes. Sprinkle with chopped coriander and serve with salad leaves.

VEGETABLE CHILLI

SERVES 4

220g/7¾oz/heaped 1 cup brown rice

4 tsp olive oil

1 onion, chopped

2 garlic cloves, crushed

4 tsp ground cumin

1 tsp chilli flakes

2 carrots, diced

4 celery sticks, diced

3 red peppers, deseeded and diced

400g/14oz/2 cups tinned red kidney beans (no added salt), rinsed and drained

800g/1lb 12oz/3⅓ cups tinned chopped tomatoes

juice of 2 lemons

1 Rinse the rice under cold running water, then put it in a saucepan and cover with cold water. Bring to the boil, then turn the heat down to medium and simmer for 35 minutes or until soft, or according to the packet instructions.

2 Heat the oil in a deep, nonstick saucepan over medium heat. Add the onion and garlic and cook for 2–3 minutes until golden. Add the cumin and chilli flakes and cook for a further 30 seconds to release the flavours. Add the carrots, celery and peppers and fry for a further 2 minutes, stirring constantly.

3 Add the kidney beans and tomatoes. Bring to the boil over high heat, then turn the heat down and simmer for 15–20 minutes until all the vegetables are tender. Stir in the lemon juice. Serve the chilli on a bed of rice.

VEGETABLE BROTH

SERVES 1

1 tsp olive oil

1 carrot, chopped

½ red pepper, deseeded and chopped

½ green pepper, deseeded and chopped

½ courgette, chopped

¼ onion, chopped

¼ garlic clove, crushed

400ml/14fl oz/scant 1⅔ cups low-sodium vegetable stock

5 green beans

2 tbsp chopped thyme leaves

salt and freshly ground black pepper

1 tsp chopped herbs (such as parsley, chervil, coriander or chives), to serve

1 Heat the oil in a saucepan over medium heat. Add the carrot, peppers, courgette, onion and garlic, reduce the heat to very low, cover with a lid and cook for about 5 minutes.

2 Add the stock and bring to the boil over high heat, then lower the heat, cover again with a lid and leave to simmer for a further 15 minutes. Add the green beans and thyme and cook for 5 minutes or until the vegetables are tender. Season to taste with salt and pepper, and sprinkle with herbs and serve.

250-CALORIE DINNERS

Try these suggestions for delicious light dinners:

- 175g/6oz skinless and boneless chicken strips, grilled, with a large green salad dressed with 1 tsp olive oil and 1 tsp balsamic vinegar.

- 175g/6oz skinless and boneless chicken breast, marinated in 1 tsp lemon juice, ¼ tsp dried thyme and pepper, then grilled. Serve with 100g/3½oz steamed mangetout.

- Chicken fajita made with 1 whole-wheat tortilla, 90g/3¼oz skinless and boneless chicken breast cut into strips and coated in a pinch of chilli and garlic powder and grilled, served with 1 sliced tomato and 1 handful of rocket leaves.

- One boneless pork loin chop, marinated in 1 tbsp lime juice, 1 tsp honey, ½ tsp cumin and 1 tsp sesame oil, then pan-fried with ½ chopped onion and served with 6 cherry tomatoes.

- 140g/5oz lean steak, 4 broccoli florets, 4 baby corn, ½ clove crushed garlic and fresh root ginger, stir-fried in 1 tbsp oyster sauce.

- 175g/6oz white fish fillet baked with a dressing of a pinch of cayenne pepper, 1 tbsp lime juice, ½ tsp crushed cumin seeds and 1 tbsp fresh coriander. Serve with 165g/5¾oz steamed vegetables of your choice.

- 175g/6oz grilled white fish fillet spread with 1 tbsp reduced-fat mayonnaise mixed with a squeeze of lemon juice and a pinch of Italian herbs. Serve with a large green salad dressed with 1 tsp olive oil and 1 tsp balsamic vinegar.

- 175g/6oz lemon sole, pan-fried in 2 tsp olive oil, served with 1 sliced green pepper, 5 cherry tomatoes, ½ clove crushed garlic and 1 tbsp chopped basil leaves.

- 120g/4¼oz salmon, grilled, then sprinkled with 1 tsp low-sodium soy sauce, served with 165g/5¾oz steamed green vegetables.

- 140g/5oz tuna steak pan-fried in 1 tsp olive oil, served on a bed of wilted spinach with a squeeze of lemon juice.

- 1 sliced red pepper and 1 large handful of spinach, stir-fried with garlic, 1 spring onion, 2 tsp soy sauce, 2 tsp sesame oil and 120g/4¼oz king prawns.

- 300ml/10½fl oz/scant 1¼ cups shop-bought lentil soup sprinkled with parsley and served with a large green salad dressed with lemon juice and black pepper.

- 2 poached eggs and 2 grilled tomatoes on a bed of wilted spinach. Season with plenty of black pepper and serve with 1 oatcake.

- 200g/7oz tofu, marinated in 2 tsp olive oil, ½ clove crushed garlic and 1 tsp paprika, baked in the oven and served with a green salad dressed with 1 tsp olive oil and 1 tsp balsamic vinegar.

- 50g/1¾oz whole-wheat spaghetti cooked and tossed with 2 tsp olive oil, ½ clove crushed garlic, 1 tbsp basil, 5 asparagus stalks and 4 halved cherry tomatoes.

- Omelette made with 2 eggs and 1 small handful of fresh baby spinach, and seasoned with salt and pepper. Serve with a tomato and onion salad drizzled with 1 tsp olive oil.

SNACKS

RAW POWER

- Choose a handful of vegetable sticks (such as pepper, carrot, courgette and cucumber) and serve with 1 heaped tbsp guacamole, hummus or other dip of your choice.

- Alternatively, if you feel like something fruity, eat a small fruit salad or 1 whole fruit (however, anything super-sweet like grapes and pineapple is generally best avoided).

PROTEIN PICK-ME-UPS

A protein-rich snack will help to prevent cravings. Simple often works best, but experiment to find what suits you. Here are some suggestions:

- 1 boiled egg.

- 3 tbsp cottage cheese, served with raw veggie dippers.

- 1 tbsp peanut butter spread on celery or sliced apple.

- 15 almonds.

- 125g/4½oz/½ cup fat-free Greek yogurt or natural yogurt. Top with some chopped fruit, if you like.

- 80g/2¾oz/1½ cups shelled edamame (soya) beans (can be bought frozen and defrosted), cooked in boiling water or steamed for 3–4 minutes until soft.

- 90g/3¼oz tinned tuna in spring water, served with 1 rice cake or oatcake.

JUICES

PINEAPPLE AND PEAR   SERVES 1

1 pear, cored and quartered
1 apple, cored and quartered
1 slice of pineapple, peeled, including
   the core

1 Put all the ingredients through
   an electric juicer, then serve.

APPLE TROPICS   SERVES 1

½ passionfruit
2 apples, cored and quartered
¼ pineapple, peeled and cut into
   chunks, including the core
1 tsp lime juice

1 Scoop out the pulp and seeds
   from the passionfruit into a
   small bowl.
2 Put the apples and pineapple
   through an electric juicer.
3 Pour the juice into a blender
   or food processor and add the
   passionfruit and lime juice.
   Process until smooth, then serve.

APPLE BLUSH   SERVES 1

1½ apples, cored and quartered
1 nectarine, stoned
4 strawberries, hulled

1 Put the apples through an
   electric juicer.
2 Pour the juice into a blender
   or food processor and add the
   nectarine and strawberries.
   Process until smooth, then serve.

ST CLEMENT'S SERVES 1

1 orange, peeled and quartered
1 grapefruit, peeled and quartered
½ lemon, peeled

1 Put all the ingredients through
   an electric juicer, then serve.

GRAPEFRUIT AND LIME SERVES 1

1½ pink grapefruits, peeled and
   quartered
1 lime, peeled

1 Put the ingredients through
   an electric juicer, then serve.

FLORIDA BLUE SERVES 1

1 orange, peeled and quartered
½ pink grapefruit, peeled and cut
   in half
1 small handful of blueberries

1 Put the orange and grapefruit
   through an electric juicer.
2 Pour the juice into a blender or
   food processor and add the
   blueberries. Process until smooth,
   then serve.

POWER-PACKED C SERVES 1

1 large orange, peeled and quartered
1 guava, peeled and chopped
5 strawberries, hulled

1 Put the orange through an electric juicer.
2 Pour the juice into a blender or food processor and add the guava and strawberries. Process until smooth, then serve.

WARM STRAWBERRY SPICE SERVES 1

1 apple, cored and quartered
1 pear, cored and quartered
6 strawberries, hulled
a pinch of mixed spice

1 Put the apple and pear through an electric juicer.
2 Pour the juice into a blender or food processor and add the strawberries. Process until smooth.
3 Pour the mixture into a saucepan, then stir in the mixed spice and heat over low heat until the juice is warm, then serve.

WARM MELON AND GINGER SERVES 1

¼ papaya, peeled, deseeded and
   chopped into chunks
1 pear, cored and quartered
¼ honeydew melon, peeled and
   deseeded
1cm/½in piece of fresh root ginger,
   peeled
a little mineral water, if needed

1 Put all the ingredients, except
the mineral water, through an
electric juicer.
2 Alternatively, put the ingredients
in a blender or food processor
and add a splash of mineral
water. Process until smooth,
and add a little more water if
necessary.
3 Pour the juice or blended mixture
into a saucepan and heat gently
over low heat until the juice is
warm, then serve.

ULTIMATE LIVER LOVER SERVES 1

4 apples
1 orange, peeled
1 lemon or lime, peeled
1cm/½in piece of fresh root ginger,
   peeled
2 tbsp flaxseed oil

1 Core and quarter 3 of the apples.
Peel and core the remaining
apple, then cut it into quarters.
2 Put all the ingredients, except
the oil, through an electric juicer.
Stir in the flaxseed oil and serve.

WHEATGRASS WHIP SERVES 1

2 apples, cored and quartered
½ pineapple, peeled and cut into
    chunks, including the core
1 handful of wheatgrass or 1 tsp
    wheatgrass powder

1 Put all the ingredients through
    an electric juicer. If your juicer
    can't handle wheatgrass, use
    wheatgrass powder, mixed with
    1 tablespoon water, and stir it
    into the juice. Serve.

DIGESTION DELIGHT SERVES 1

3 carrots, unpeeled
½ pineapple, peeled and cut into
    chunks, including the core
1 small handful of strawberries
½ papaya, peeled, deseeded and
    chopped into chunks

1 Put the carrots and pineapple
    through an electric juicer.
2 Pour the juice into a blender
    or food processor and add the
    strawberries and papaya.
    Process until smooth, then serve.

GUT SOOTHER SERVES 1

1 pear, cored and quartered
1 carrot, unpeeled
¼ pineapple, peeled and cut into
    chunks, including the core
1.5cm/⅝in piece of fresh root ginger,
    peeled

1 Put all the ingredients through
    an electric juicer, then serve.

JUMP-OUT-OF-BED JUICE SERVES 1

4 carrots, unpeeled
2 apples, cored and quartered
½ pineapple, peeled and cut into
   chunks, including the core

1 Put all the ingredients through
an electric juicer, then serve.

PASSION SERVES 1

1 passionfruit
3 oranges, peeled and quartered
½ lime, peeled
2 carrots, unpeeled

1 Cut the passionfruit in half and
scoop out the pulp and seeds
into a small bowl.
2 Put all the ingredients through
an electric juicer, then serve.

APPLE ZING SERVES 1

1 apple, cored and quartered
1 carrot, unpeeled
5mm/¼in piece of fresh root ginger,
   peeled

1 Put all the ingredients through
an electric juicer, then serve.

COOLING CUCUMBER SERVES 1

½ cucumber

1 apple, cored and quartered

1 Peel the cucumber if you would like a sweeter flavour.

2 Put the ingredients through an electric juicer, then serve.

VEGGIE APPLE MAGIC SERVES 1

½ small cucumber

4 carrots, unpeeled

2 celery sticks

1 apple, cored and quartered

1 Peel the cucumber if you would like a sweeter flavour.

2 Put all the ingredients through an electric juicer, then serve.

GRAPE CRUNCH SERVES 1

2 celery sticks

25 red grapes

1 Put the ingredients through an electric juicer, then serve.

GOLDEN CARROT SERVES 1

1 small orange, peeled and halved
½ lime, peeled
1cm/½in piece of fresh root ginger,
    peeled
1 small apple, cored and quartered
2 large carrots, unpeeled

1 Put all the ingredients through
  an electric juicer, then serve.

MINT MEDLEY SERVES 1

¼ pineapple, peeled and cut into
    chunks, including the core
1cm/½in piece of fresh root ginger,
    peeled
½ thick slice of white cabbage
1 small handful of mint leaves

1 Put all the ingredients through
  an electric juicer, then serve.

POPEYE SERVES 1

¼ cucumber
1 handful of baby spinach
1 apple, cored and quartered
½ pineapple, peeled and cut into
    chunks, including the core
1 lime, peeled

1 Peel the cucumber if you would
  like a sweeter flavour.
2 Put all the ingredients through
  an electric juicer, then serve.

CARROT CUP SERVES 1

1 small handful of coriander leaves

3 large carrots, unpeeled

1 Put the coriander through an electric juicer, then push the carrots through, and serve.

CARROT AND CELERY SERVES 1

2 large carrots, unpeeled

3 celery sticks

1 Put the ingredients through an electric juicer, then serve.

CARROT AND BEETROOT SERVES 1

2 large carrots, unpeeled, cut into chunks

⅓ raw beetroot, unpeeled, cut into chunks

2 tbsp fresh basil leaves

1 Put the basil between the chunks of carrot and beetroot and push through an electric juicer. Serve.

GREEN WONDER SERVES

1 celery stick
6 kale leaves
2 tomatoes
1 tbsp oregano leaves (optional)
½ ripe avocado, peeled, pitted and mashed

1 Put the celery, kale, tomatoes and oregano, if using, through an electric juicer.
2 Pour the juice into a blender or food processor and add the avocado. Process until smooth, then serve.

VEGGIE COCKTAIL SERVES 1

1 celery stick
2 tomatoes
1 carrot, unpeeled
¼ lemon, peeled

1 Put all the ingredients through an electric juicer, then serve.

A FINAL WORD

If you've read this book and are still trying to decide if, when or how to give fasting a try, stop! Don't intellectualize or rationalize it. You'll only ever truly "get it" by trying for yourself.

It is a leap of faith to believe that something as simple as drinking juice can do what pills and potions cannot. **So, you just need to make the leap and see what happens.**

You need to remember that **healing from the inside is something your body is *designed* to do.** If you create the right conditions, the body will respond. **Fasting can create the right internal environment for healing and positive change to occur.**

The same process happens emotionally, too. There is nothing quite like the perspective or creative leap that occurs in the mind when you take time out from your norm. **Just imagine what life could be like if you followed your dreams.**

I know because that is exactly what happened to me. Before I end this book I want to tell you the story of the TV series that first spread the word of the power of fasting. It's something I am asked about all the time, all over the world, and it's a story I've never told fully before now.

I admitted at the beginning of the book that I kind of stumbled upon fasting. I had already studied Nutritional Medicine so I had a good grounding in the science of sound eating. However, when I started using juice fasting, first on my own and then with clients, the results were so astonishing that it was the push I needed to give up a six-figure salary, sell a house and drive to Spain with nothing more than the notion of following my dream to set up my first juice-fasting retreat.

One year later I had learned the local lingo, made lifelong friends and was enjoying a wonderful lifestyle of yoga on the beach, tapas and siestas. Alas, my dwindling bank balance told a different story. I had hired a rustic villa in the mountains to run juice retreats for a few people at a time, working from dawn till dusk and doing everything myself – not exactly a sustainable business model.

A random email from an old TV contact was the reality check I needed to put the retreats – and fasting – on the map. I worked up a pitch document and decided to knock on the doors of any media person I knew to get the format made into a TV series. Thirteen knock-backs later and I finally got a "yes".

My retreats ended up becoming the subject of more than seven TV series, shown in over 22 countries around the world, which continue to be shown today.

I believe that the reason the series became such a phenomenon is that it showed, beyond a shadow of a doubt, that even dramatic health conditions are curable.

Almost a decade on, I still have people from all over the world getting in touch or attending my retreats who say that watching the series gave them hope and a new direction. Many times over I've been told that seeing health transformed using something as simple as a fast was the nudge they needed to take action in their own lives.

GLOSSARY

Adrenals A pair of glands found on top of the kidneys that produce hormones involved in regulating fluid balance, metabolism and the body's response to stress.

Alzheimer's The most common type of dementia, a brain disease that leads to progressive memory loss along with mood and personality changes.

Amino acids Tiny molecules that are the building blocks of proteins. We obtain them from protein-rich foods and then use them for growth and repair and to make enzymes, hormones and antibodies.

Antioxidant Substances found in food (for example, vitamin C) or made by the body that help protect cells from free radical damage.

Autophagy A process that enables your cells to identify and break down damaged components – like spring cleaning for the body.

Beta-oxidation The process of breaking down fatty acids (molecules of fat) to release energy.

Bile An alkaline fluid made by the liver and stored in the gallbladder, which is then released into the intestine to aid the absorption of fats.

Carbohydrates (carbs)) Nutrients made from chains of individual sugar molecules. Usually referred to as either simple or complex. Complex carbohydrates are long chains that tend to be more slowly absorbed.

Catecholamines Neurotransmitter molecules that help the body respond to stress.

Cholesterol A substance with many roles, including the synthesis of cell membranes, hormones and vitamin D. High levels of the oxidized form of the cholesterol transport protein LDL are associated with blood vessel damage.

Cortisol A hormone released by the adrenals in response to stress. It stimulates the release of sugars into the bloodstream.

CRP (C-Reactive Protein) A protein made by the liver that is found in high levels when the body is experiencing inflammation.

Cytokines Proteins involved in the regulation of immunity and inflammation.

DNA The "instructions" found in every cell that determine our individual characteristics. The cells use these instructions to make new proteins.

Essential fatty acids (EFAs) These fatty acids, such as omega-3, can't be synthesized inside the body, so must be obtained from the diet.

Estradiol A natural form of oestrogen secreted by the ovaries. It has a number of roles in female fertility, including triggering ovulation.

Follicle stimulating hormone (FSH) A hormone produced in the brain that stimulates the ovary to mature an egg.

Free radicals An unstable molecule, produced either through normal biological processes (including breathing) or from toxins such as smoke. Unless neutralized by an antioxidant, it can damage the cells.

Ghrelin A hormone secreted by the stomach that stimulates the appetite.

Glucagon A hormone produced by the pancreas that promotes the breakdown and release of sugar into the bloodstream when blood sugar levels are low.

Glycogen The storage form of the sugar, *glucose*.

Glucose An individual sugar molecule. It is the preferred source of energy for the brain and red blood cells. Blood glucose levels are maintained within a narrow range.

Growth hormone (GH) A hormone produced in the brain that regulates growth.

High-density lipoprotein (HDL) Often referred to as "good" *cholesterol*, this is a transport protein that helps transport excess cholesterol out of the bloodstream.

Hormone A substance made in one part of the body that triggers a reaction in another part of the body.

Hypothalamus An area of the brain that controls body temperature, hunger, thirst and fatigue.

IL-6 A protein involved in the regulation of the immune system and inflammation.

Insulin A hormone produced by the pancreas that promotes the storage of sugar, protein and fat when blood sugar levels are raised.

Insulin-like growth factor (IGF-1) A hormone similar to *insulin* that plays a role in growth.

Ketone bodies Substances synthesized from fats when *carbohydrate* intake is low. They can be used as an alternative form of fuel by the cells, including the brain.

Laron Syndrome A hereditary condition that prevents the body from growing normally. It is associated with low levels of *IGF-1*.

Leptin A hormone produced from the fat cells, which reduces appetite.

Lipase Enzymes involved in the breakdown of fats.

Lipolysis A process through which the body breaks down fats.

Luteinizing hormone (LH) A hormone produced in the brain that stimulates ovulation.

Mitochondria The cells' energy-producing powerhouses.

Oestrogen Any of a group of hormones that have a number of roles in the female body, including involvement in sexual development, ovulation and pregnancy.

Parkinson's A degenerative disease of the central nervous system that affects movement patterns and can progress to affect cognitive function.

Progesterone A hormone secreted by the ovary that thickens the womb lining.

Serotonin A "feelgood" neurotransmitter found primarily in the brain.

Stroke The obstruction of a blood vessel in the brain.

Thermogenesis The production of heat within the body.

TNFa A protein involved in the body's response to inflammation.

Triglycerides Fats made up of groups of three fatty acids.

BIBLIOGRAPHY

OVERVIEWS OF THE RESEARCH ON WEIGHT AND HEALTH
Butland, B. *et al.* (2007) *Foresight, Tackling Obesities: Future Choices – Project report.*
London: Department of Innovation Universities and Skills.

Song, X. *et al.* (2012) Relationship between body mass index and mortality among
Europeans. European Journal of Clinical Nutrition, 66:156–165.

WEIGHT GAIN CAN BE CATCHING!
Christakis, N.A. and Fowler, J.H. (2007) The spread of obesity in a large social network
over 32 years. *New England Journal of Medicine, 357:* 370–379.

HOW EXTERNAL FACTORS AFFECT WEIGHT
Swinburn, B. *et al.* (1999) Dissecting obesogenic environments: the development and
application of a framework for identifying and prioritising environmental interventions
for obesity. *Preventive Medicine, 29*(6):563–570.

HOW SNACKING AFFECTS WEIGHT
Berteus-Forslund, H. *et al.* (2005) Snacking frequency in relation to energy intake and
food choices in obese men and women compared to reference population. *International
Journal of Obesity*, 29(6):711–719.

HOW SLEEP AFFECTS WEIGHT
Cappuccio, FP *et al.* (2008) Meta analysis of short sleep duration and obesity in
children and adults. *Sleep, 31*(5):619–626.

Knutson, K.L. (2012) Does inadequate sleep play a role in vulnerability to obesity?
American Journal of Human Biology, 24:361–371.

HOW ALCOHOL AFFECTS FAT METABOLISM
Siler, S.Q., Neese, R.A., and Hellerstein, M.K. (1999). De-novo lipogenesis, lipid
kinetics, and whole-body lipid balances in humans after acute alcohol consumption.
American Journal of Clinical Nutrition, 70:928–936.

RESEARCH ON THE MEASUREMENT OF OBESITY
Romero-Corral, A. *et al.* (2008) Accuracy of Body Mass Index to Diagnose Obesity in
the US Adult Population. *International Journal of Obesity, 32*(6):959–966.

WHY IT CAN BE DIFFICULT TO LOSE WEIGHT AND KEEP IT OFF LONG-TERM
Hall, K.D. *et al.* (2011) Quantification of the effect of energy imbalance on bodyweight.
The Lancet, 378:826–837.

Sumithran, P. *et al.* (2011) Long-term persistence of hormonal adaptations to weight loss. *New England Journal of Medicine*, 365:1597–1604.

THE EFFECTS OF YO-YO DIETING ON WEIGHT
Mason, C. *et al.* (2012) History of weight cycling does not impede future weight loss or metabolic improvements in postmenopausal women. *Metabolism – Clinical and Experimental*, 62(1):127–136.

WHICH IS MORE IMPORTANT FOR WEIGHT LOSS – DIET OR EXERCISE?
Tsai, A.C., Sandretto, A. and Chung, Y.C. (2003) Dieting is more effective in reducing weight but exercise is more effective in reducing fat during the early phase of a weight-reducing program in healthy humans. *Journal of Nutritional Biochemistry,* 14(9):541–549.

MEDICAL WEIGHT MANAGEMENT GUIDELINES
Scottish Intercollegiate Guidelines Network (2010) *Management of obesity.* Scottish Intercollegiate Guidelines Network, Edinburgh.

HEALTH STATISTICS
Centers for Disease Control and Prevention (2011) *Diagnosed and undiagnosed diabetes in the United States, all ages, 2010* [online] Available from: http: //www.cdc.gov/diabetes/pubs/estimates11.htm#1 [last accessed 31/10/12].

Diabetes U.K. (2012) *Diabetes in the U.K. 2012* [online] Available from: http: //www.diabetes.org.uk/Documents/Reports/Diabetes-in-the-UK-2012.pdf [last accessed 31/10/12].

Hippisley-Cox, J. and Coupland, C. (2012) Unintended effects of statins in men and women in England and Wales: a population based cohort study using the QResearch database. *British Medical Journal,* 340:c2197.

The Information Centre (2008) *Prescriptions Dispensed in the Community: Statistics for 1997 to 2007: England* [online] Available from: http: //www.ic.nhs.uk/webfiles/publications/PCA%20publication/Final%20version%20210708.pdf [last accessed 31/10/12]

World Health Organization (2012) *World Health Statistics 2012* [online] Available from: http: //www.who.int/healthinfo/EN_WHS2012_Full.pdf [last accessed 31/10/12]

HOW CHANGING MEAL FREQUENCY AFFECTS HORMONES, BLOOD SUGAR AND APPETITE
Alken, J., Petriczko, E. and Marcus, C. (2008) Effect of fasting on young adults who have symptoms of hypoglycaemia in the absence of frequent meals. *European Journal of Clinical Nutrition*, 62(56):721–726.

Bogdan, A., Bouchareb, B. and Touitou, Y. (2005) Response of circulating leptin to Ramadan daytime fasting: a circadian study. *British Journal of Nutrition, 93*(4):515–518.

Boyle, P.J., Shah, S.D. and Cryer, P.E. (1989) Insulin, glucagon and catecholamines in prevention of hypoglycaemia during fasting. *American Journal of Physiology, 256*(5 Pt 1): E651–661.

Frecka, J.M. and Mattes, R.D. (2008) Possible entrainment of ghrelin to habitual meal patterns in humans. *American Journal of Physiology: Gastrointestinal and Liver Physiology*, 294(3)G699–G707.

Johnstone, A.M. *et al.* (2002) Effect of an acute fast on energy compensation and feeding behaviour in lean men and women. *International Journal of Obesity, 26*:1623–1628.

Kolaczynski, J.W. *et al.* (1996) Responses of leptin to short-term fasting and refeeding in humans: a link with ketogenesis but not ketones themselves. *Diabetes, 45*(11):1511–1515.

Leidy, H.J. and Campbell, W.W. (2011) The effect of eating frequency on appetite control and food intake: brief synopsis of controlled feeding studies. *The Journal of Nutrition, 141*:154s–157s.

Stote, K.S. *et al.* (2007) A controlled trial of reduced meal frequency without calorie restriction in healthy, normal-weight, middle-aged adults. *American Journal of Clinical Nutrition, 85*(4):981–988.

IS INTERMITTENT FASTING MORE EFFECTIVE THAN CALORIE COUNTING?
Harvie, M.N. *et al.* (2011) The effects of intermittent or continuous energy restriction on weight loss and metabolic disease risk markers: a randomised trial in young overweight women. *International Journal of Obesity, 35*(5):714–727.

Varady, K.A. (2011) Intermittent versus daily calorie restriction: which diet regimen is more effective for weight loss? *Obesity Reviews, 12*:e593–e601.

HOW FASTING AFFECTS YOUR METABOLIC RATE
Mansell, P.L., Fellows, I.W. and MacDonald, I.A. (1990) Enhanced thermogenic response to epinephrine after 48-h starvation in humans. *American Journal of Physiology, 258*(1 Pt 2):R87–93.

Martin, A. *et al.* (2000) Is advice for breakfast consumption justified? Results from a short-term dietary and metabolic experiment in young healthy men. *British Journal of Nutrition, 84*(3):337–344.

Webber, J. and Macdonald, I.A. (1994) The cardiovascular, metabolic and hormonal changes accompanying acute starvation in men and women. *British Journal of Nutrition, 71*(3):434–447.

FASTING FOR FAT LOSS

Helibronn, L.K. *et al.* (2005) Alternate-day fasting in nonobese subjects: effects on body weight, body composition and energy metabolism. *American Journal of Clinical Nutrition*, 81:69–73.

THE EFFECTS OF FASTING ON PEOPLE OF DIFFERENT WEIGHTS

Elia, M., Stubbs, R.J. and Henry, C.J.K. (1999) Differences in fat, carbohydrate and protein metabolism between lean and obese subjects undergoing total starvation. *Obesity Research*, 7(6):597–604.

OVERVIEW OF THE RESEARCH ON FASTING AND HEALTH

Johnstone, A.M. (2007) Fasting – the ultimate diet? *Obesity Reviews*, 8:211–222.

HOW FASTING AFFECTS RISK FACTORS FOR HEART DISEASE AND DIABETES

Carlson, O. *et al.* (2007) Impact of Reduced Meal Frequency Without Caloric Restriction on Glucose Regulation in Healthy, Normal Weight Middle-Aged Men and Women. *Metabolism*, 56(12):1729–1734.

Gomez, J.C. (2011) *Press release: Study finds routine periodic fasting is good for your health, and your heart.* [online] Available from: http: //www.eurekalert.org/pub_releases/2011-04/imc-sfr033111.php [last accessed: 30/10/2012].

Halberg, N. *et al.* (2005) Effect of intermittent fasting and refeeding on insulin action in healthy men. *Journal of Applied Physiology*, 99 (6):2128–2136.

Harvie, M.N. *et al.* (2011) The effects of intermittent or continuous energy restriction on weight loss and metabolic disease risk markers: a randomised trial in young overweight women. *International Journal of Obesity*, 35(5):714–727.

Heilbronn, L.K. *et al.* (2005) Glucose tolerance and skeletal muscle gene expression in response to alternate day fasting. *Obesity Research*, 13(3):574–581.

Varady, K.A. *et al.* (2009) Short-term modified alternate-day fasting: a novel dietary strategy for weight loss and cardioprotection in obese adults. *American Journal of Clinical Nutrition*, 90(5):1138–1143.

Wing, R.R. *et al.* (1994) Year-long weight loss treatment for obese patients with type II diabetes: Does including an intermittent very-low-calorie diet improve outcome? *The American Journal of Medicine*, 97(4):354–362.

FASTING AND AUTOPHAGY

Alirezaei, M. *et al.* (2010) Short-term fasting induces profound neuronal autophagy. *Autophagy*, 6(6): 702–710.

HOW RESTRICTING CALORIES OR FASTING MAY HELP PREVENT OR TREAT CANCER

Fontana, L. (2008) Long-term effects of calorie or protein restriction on serum IGF-1 and IGFBP-3 concentration in humans. *Aging Cell,* 7(5):681–687.

Johnson, J.B. (2008) Pretreatment with alternate day modified fast will permit higher dose and frequency of cancer chemotherapy and better cure rates. *Medical Hypotheses,* 72(4):381–382.

Lee, C. *et al.* (2012) Fasting cycles retard growth of tumors and sensitize a range of cancer cell types to chemotherapy. *Science Translational Medicine,* 4(124):124.

Longo, V.D. and Fontana, L. (2010) Calorie restriction and cancer prevention: metabolic and molecular mechanisms. *Trends in Pharmacological Science,* 31(2):89–98.

Safdie, F.M. *et al.* (2009) Fasting and cancer treatment in humans: a case series report. *Aging,* 1(12):988–1007.

THE CANCER-FIGHTING PROPERTIES OF GREEN TEA

Komori, A. *et al.* (1993) Anticarcinogenic activity of green tea polyphenols. *Japan Journal of Clinical Oncology,* 23(3).

HOW FASTING AFFECTS INFLAMMATION

Aksungar, F.B., Topkaya, A.E. and Akyildiz, M. (2007) Interleukin-6, C-reactive protein and biochemical parameters during prolonged intermittent fasting. *Annals of Nutrition and Metabolism,* 51(1):88–95.

Dixit, V.D. *et al.* (2011) Controlled meal frequency without caloric restriction alters peripheral blood mononuclear cell cytokine production. *Journal of Inflammation,* 8:6.

Johnson, J.B. *et al.* (2007) Alternate day calorie restriction improves clinical findings and reduces markers of oxidative stress and inflammation in overweight adults with moderate asthma. *Free Radical Biology and Medicine,* 42(5):665–674.

HOW FASTING AFFECTS FEMALE HORMONES

Alvero, R. *et al.* (1998) Effects of fasting on neuroendocrine function and follicle development in lean women. *Journal of Clinical Endocrinology and Metabolism,* 83:76–80.

Bergendahl, M. *et al.* (1999) Short-term fasting suppresses leptin and (conversely) activates disorderly growth hormone secretion in midluteal phase women – a clinical research center study. *The Journal of Clinical Endocrinology and Metabolism,* 84(3):883–894.

Hartman, M.L. *et al.* (1992) Augmented growth hormone (GH) secretory burst frequency and amplitude mediate enhanced GH secretion during a two-day fast in normal men. *The Journal of Clinical Endocrinology and Metabolism,* 74(4):757–765.

Martin, B. *et al.* (2007) Sex-dependent metabolic, neuroendocrine and cognitive responses to dietary energy restriction and excess. *Endocrinology, 148*(9):4318–4333.

Soules, M.R. *et al.* (1994) Short-term fasting in normal women: absence of effect on gonadotrophin secretion and the menstrual cycle. *Clinical Endocrinology, 40*(6):725–731.

HOW THE MENSTRUAL CYCLE AFFECTS APPETITE
McNeil, J. and Doucet, E. (2012) Possible factors for altered energy balance across the menstrual cycle: a closer look at the severity of PMS, reward driven behaviours and leptin variations. *European Journal of Obstetrics and Reproductive Biology, 163*(1):5–10.

THE ROLE OF GROWTH HORMONE IN MAINTAINING MUSCLE MASS
Kanaley, J.A. *et al.* (1997) Human growth hormone response to repeated bouts of aerobic exercise. *Journal of Applied Physiology, 83*(5):1756–1761.

Moller, N. *et al.* (2009) Growth hormone and protein metabolism. *Clinical Nutrition, 28*(6):597–603.

Norrelund, H. *et al.* (2001) The protein-retaining effects of growth hormone during fasting involve inhibition of muscle-protein breakdown. *Diabetes, 50*(1):96–104.

PROTEIN AND BELLY FAT
Loenneke, J.P. *et al.* (2012) Quality protein is inversely related with abdominal fat. *Nutrition and Metabolism, 9*(1):5.

HOW MUCH EXERCISE DO YOU NEED?
World Health Organization (2010) *Global Recommendations on Physical Activity for Health.* Available at: http://whqlibdoc.who.int/publications/2010/9789241599979_eng.pdf

DOES EXERCISING WHILE FASTED AFFECT PERFORMANCE?
Chaouachi, A. *et al.* (2012) The effects of Ramadan intermittent fasting on athletic performance: Recommendations for the maintenance of physical fitness. *Journal of Sports Sciences, 30*(s1):S53–73.

Ferguson, L.M. *et al.* (2009) Effects of caloric restriction and overnight fasting on cycling endurance performance. *Journal of Strength and Conditioning Research, 23*(2):560–570.

Schisler, J.A. and Ianuzzo, C.D. (2007) Running to maintain cardiovascular fitness is not limited by short-term fasting or enhanced by carbohydrate supplementation. *Journal of Physical Activity and Health, 4*(1):101–112.

THE EFFECTS OF EXERCISING FASTED ON METABOLISM
Farah, N.M.F. and Gill, J.M.R. (2012) Effects of exercise before or after meal ingestion

on fat balance and prostprandial metabolism in overweight men. *British Journal of Nutrition*, doi: 10.1017/S0007114512004448.

Hulston, C.J. *et al.* (2010) Training with low muscle glycogen enhances fat metabolism in well-trained cyclists. *Medicine and Science in Sports and Exercise*, 42(11):2046–2055.

Knapik, J.J. *et al.* (1988) Influence of fasting on carbohydrate and fat metabolism during rest and exercise in men. *Journal of Applied Physiology,* 64(5):1923–1929.

Trabelski, K. *et al.* (2012) Effects of fed- versus fasted-state aerobic training during Ramadan on body composition and some metabolic parameters in physically active men. *International Journal of Sports Nutrition and Exercise Metabolism, 22*(1):11–18.

THE EFFECTS OF EXERCISING FASTED OR FED ON MUSCLES
Civitarese, A.E. *et al.* (2005) Glucose ingestion during exercise blunts exercise-induced gene expression of skeletal muscle oxidative genes. *American Journal of Physiology – Endocrinology and Metabolism, 289*:e1023–e1029.

Deldicque, L. *et al.* (2010) Increased $p70^{s6k}$ phosphorylation during intake of a protein-carbohydrate drink following resistance training in the fasted state. *European Journal of Applied Physiology, 108*(4):791–800.

Psilander, N. *et al.* (2012) Exercise with low glycogen increases PGC-1a gene expression in human skeletal muscle. *European Journal of Applied Physiology*, PMID: 23053125.

Stannard, S.R. *et al.* (2010) Adaptations to skeletal muscle with endurance exercise training in the acutely fed versus overnight fasted state. *Journal of Science and Medicine in Sport, 13*:465–469.

THE EFFECTS OF FASTING ON BALANCE
Johnson, S. and Leck, K. (2010) The effects of dietary fasting on physical balance among healthy young women. *Nutrition Journal, 9*:18.

HOW FASTING AFFECTS THE BRAIN
Halagappa, V.K. *et al.* (2007) Intermittent fasting and caloric restriction ameliorate age-related behavioral deficits in the triple-transgenic mouse model of Alzheimer's disease. *Neurobiology of Disease, 26*(1):212–220.

Kramer, A.F., Erickson, K.I. and Colcombe, S.J. (2006) Exercise, cognition, and the aging brain/*Journal of Applied Physiology*, 101(4):1237–1242.

Lieberman, H.R. (2008) A double-blind, placebo-controlled test of 2 d of calorie deprivation: effects on cognition, activity, sleep, and interstitial glucose concentrations. *American Journal of Clinical Nutrition, 88*:667–676.

Martin, B., Mattson, M.P. and Maudsley, S. (2006) Caloric restriction and intermittent fasting: two potential diets for successful brain aging. *Ageing Research Reviews,* 5(3):332–353.

Middleton, L.E. *et al.* (2011) Activity Energy Expenditure and Incident Cognitive Impairment in Older Adults. *Archives of Internal Medicine,* 171(14):1251–1257.

Rothman, S.M. and Mattson, M.P. (2012) Activity-dependent, stress-responsive BDNF signaling and the quest for optimal brain health and resilience throughout the lifespan. *Neuroscience,* 10.1016/j.neuroscience.2012.10.014. [Epub ahead of print].

Vercambre, M.N. *et al.* (2011) Physical activity and cognition in women with vascular conditions. *Archives of Internal Medicine,* 171(14):1244–1250.

THE EFFECTS OF FASTING ON LIFESPAN

Johnson, J.B. (2006) The effect on health of alternate day calorie restriction: Eating less and more than needed on alternate days prolongs life. *Medical Hypotheses,* 67(2):209–211.

Trepanowski, J. (2011) Impact of caloric and dietary restriction regimens on markers of health and longevity in humans and animals: a summary of available findings. *Nutrition Journal,* 10:107.

A PRACTICAL GUIDE TO HELP YOU AVOID OVER-THINKING THINGS

Newbigging, S. (2012) THUNK! *How to Think Less for Serenity and Success.* Findhorn Press, Forres.

BEING SMART DOESN'T MEAN YOU HAVE MORE WILLPOWER

Shiv, B. and Fedorikhin, A. (1999) Heart and mind in conflict: the interplay of affect and cognition in consumer decision making. *Journal of Consumer Research,* 26(3): 278–292.

WHY IT'S IMPORTANT TO PLAN YOUR FIRST MEAL AFTER A FAST

Goldstone, T. (2012) *Good Breakfast and Good Diet: New Findings Support Common Sense.* [online] available from: http: //www.sfn.org/am2012/pdf/press/Diet.pdf [last accessed 30/10/2012].

Wansink, B., Tal, A. and Shimuzu, M. (2012) First foods most: after 18-hour fast, people drawn to starches first and vegetables last. *Archives of Internal Medicine,* 172(12):961–963.

INDEX

Recipes in italics feature in the fasting plans on pages 178–82

AUTHOR'S ACKNOWLEDGEMENTS

For me, this book is much more than the words on these pages. It brings together a very personal story of people and places that inspired me to follow a path without ever knowing where it would lead.

There have been several exceptional people who have been pivotal along the way and I'd like to thank them. Harry Bell and his team at Tern Television who told the story of our fasting retreats so well; Grace Cheetham at Duncan Baird for seeing the vision of the book in a few simple paragraphs and Jane for her skilled editing; my agents Jayne and Julia at Champion Talent and Borra Garson; Sarah Dempster, fellow nutritionist and academic lifeboat who has contributed above and beyond to this book; to my clients, each and every one, who always inspire me to learn more and do more; to my parents who have lovingly accepted my utter disregard for a conventional route in life; to amazing friends like Hala, Lou, Lucy and Richard who have provided space in their homes and hearts for my life out of a suitcase and most of all, to my children Hannah, Callum, Jana and Ruaridh and my husband for being simply the reason behind the reason behind the reason.

For information on any of Amanda's fasting retreats, media and books, or online weight-loss support, visit www.amandahamilton.com